Clinical Trials in Retinitis Pigmentosa Treatment

Jeffrey N. Weiss

Clinical Trials in Retinitis Pigmentosa Treatment

Springer

Jeffrey N. Weiss
Parkland, FL, USA

ISBN 978-3-031-58798-6 ISBN 978-3-031-58799-3 (eBook)
https://doi.org/10.1007/978-3-031-58799-3

This Springer imprint is published by the registered company Springer Nature Switzerland AG
The registered company address is: Gewerbestrasse 11, 6330 Cham, Switzerland

For the patients that have allowed us the privilege to serve.

Preface

This book is a compendium of the worldwide ocular stem cell, gene therapy, optogenetic, and other miscellaneous studies treating Retinitis Pigmentosa registered with Clinicaltrials.gov. Clinicaltrials.gov is the largest website listing of registered clinical research studies in the world. The information presented is accurate as of September 2023. I have divided the studies into multiple categories: Completed, Active/Recruiting, Active/Not-Recruiting, Not Yet Recruiting, and Enrolling by Invitation. Regarding study location, United States locations are listed first, followed by other countries in alphabetical order.

I have corrected the mischaracterization of studies, to only include those that truly belong within each category, and to correct spelling and grammar, while maintaining the original spirit and intent of the researchers, so as to produce a consistent and easy-to-read format. The Study title and the clinical trial number are provided in order to make it easier for the reader to obtain further information.

I hope that by providing this reference, the field of retinitis pigmentosa treatment will be advanced.

Parkland, FL, USA Jeffrey N. Weiss

Contents

Chapter 1
Introduction to Retinitis Pigmentosa

The term "retinitis pigmentosa" is generally attributed to Donders in 1855 and 1857, though evidence for its existence presumably dates back earlier to 1744 when Ovelgun reported cases of familial night blindness. The ophthalmoscope was invented by Helmholtz in 1851, and shortly thereafter, van Trigt (1853) and Ruete (1853) described cases of presumed retinitis pigmentosa (RP). The term is actually a misnomer, as inflammation is not a significant part of the condition.

RP is a spectrum, or a group of genetically determined degenerations characterized by rod dysfunction leading to cone loss. Depending on the severity of genetic expression, the patient may experience no significant symptoms, as in sector RP, or significant symptoms, such as night blindness (nyctalopia), visual field loss, loss of central vision, and blindness. The age of onset varies, depending on the type of RP, from infancy to adulthood.

Other terms have been used to describe the condition, including rod-cone dystrophy, pigmentary retinopathy, primary pigmentary retinal degeneration, and tapetoretinal degeneration. RP is the inclusive term, but subtypes such as sector RP, inverse RP, and adult-onset RP have been described.

The prevalence of RP is 1 in 3500 (US), 1 in 4016 (China), 1 in 4500 (Israel), and 1 in 7000 (Switzerland). Though RP is a genetic condition, inherited as an autosomal recessive, autosomal dominant, or as an X-linked recessive trait, from 15% to 63% of cases has no family history of the condition. An estimated two million individuals worldwide are estimated to suffer from the disease. It is the leading cause of inherited blindness.

Nyctalopia is a common symptom of this condition. In autosomal recessive RP, the median age for developing nyctalopia is 10.7 years and, in the autosomal dominant condition, 23.4 years. Dark adaptometry may demonstrate elevation of the cone segment, the rod segment, or both. There may be a delay in reaching final dark adaptation.

Progressive visual field loss, initially manifested with smaller and dimmer test objects, is noted. The earliest visual field defects are frequently relative

J. N. Weiss, *Clinical Trials in Retinitis Pigmentosa Treatment*,
https://doi.org/10.1007/978-3-031-58799-3_1

midperipheral scotomas that enlarge over time forming ring scotomas. The visual field loss corresponds closely to the fundus appearance with greater field loss in the eye with more pigmentary abnormality.

RP patients have reported photopsias in their midperipheral visual field adjacent to the areas of relative or absolute scotomas. This is presumably caused by abnormal signals from the degenerating retina. The symptoms may be confused with ophthalmic migraine but differ in that the photopsias may be continuous and are generally stationary within the field. As the scotomas increase in density, the photopsias will diminish and disappear.

The earliest funduscopic abnormalities of RP are retinal vessel attenuation and fine retinal pigment epithelial mottling in the mid and far periphery. Retinal pigment epithelial disintegration migrates into the interstitial spaces at retinal vessels producing bone-spicules and perivascular pigment cuffing. Vessel attenuation may become severe over time. Fluorescein angiography may demonstrate RPE transmission defects, diffuse leakage, and cystoid macular edema. The prevalence of cataracts in patients with RP is dependent on the genetic defect and the patient age. Posterior subcapsular cataracts are the most common type of lenticular opacity.

There are multiple syndromes associated with RP:

1. Usher's Syndrome—The most common condition consisting of RP and deafness accounting for 50% of the patients who are both deaf and blind. Usher's syndrome may be divided into Type I, Type II, and Type III. Type I is the prepubertal onset of RP and profound prelingual deafness, and Type II with more a more variable expression of RP, possibly milder, and partial deafness. Type III (Hallgren's syndrome) is characterized by congenital deafness, RP, and vestibular ataxia. There is controversy whether this is a truly separate entity from Type I. A Type IV has also been described, associated with mental retardation, but this too may not be a separate entity from the more recognized Types I and II.

Other syndromes associated with RP include:

1. Abetalipoproteinemia (Bassen–Kornzweig syndrome)
2. Alstrom's disease
3. Arteriohepatic dysplasia (Alagille syndrome, cholestasis with peripheral pulmonary stenosis)
4. Bardet–Biedl syndrome
5. Cockayne's syndrome (Neill–Dingwall syndrome)
6. Flynn–Aird syndrome
7. Hallervorden–Spatz syndrome (Neuroaxonal dystrophy, late infantile)
8. Infantile Refsum's disease (infantile phytanic acid storage disease)
9. Refsum's disease (phytanic acid oxidase deficiency)
10. Jeune's syndrome (asphyxiating thoracic dystrophy; thoracic pelvic-phalangeal dystrophy)
11. Kearns–Sayre syndrome (chronic progressive external ophthalmoplegia (CPEO) plus)
12. Laurence–Moon Hutchinson syndrome

13. Mucopolysaccharidoses
14. Neuronal ceroid lipofuscinosis (Batten's disease)
15. Late infantile form (Jansky–Bielschowsky form)
16. Juvenile (Batten–Mayou disease, Vogt–Spielmeyer disease)
17. Adult (Kufs' disease)

Differential Diagnosis of RP

Rubella retinopathy may mistakenly be diagnosed as RP, as it can cause a similar panretinal pattern. This is more likely to occur in the presence of deafness, as the child is mistakenly diagnosed with rubella retinopathy and deafness, and not RP and deafness (Usher's syndrome). A distinguishing feature is the electroretinogram (ERG) which is normal or just mildly abnormal in rubella retinopathy, but is severely abnormal in Usher's syndrome.

Syphilis, congenital or acquired, may demonstrate a pigmentary retinopathy that is similar in appearance to advanced RP. Careful examination will distinguish between the two conditions. Congenital syphilis generally includes interstitial keratitis with patchy, post-inflammatory appearing pigmentary clumps involving the posterior pole as well as the posterior fundus with a possible overlying vitreous reaction. Acquired syphilis may resemble an advanced retinal degeneration.

Infections, such as toxoplasmosis, herpes, and cytomegalovirus, may produce a retinal appearance similar to RP. However, unless the entire retina is severely damaged, the ERG will be normal or mildly abnormal. A random and patchy lesion distribution may also serve to distinguish the correct cause.

Cancer-associated retinopathy may produce extensive panretinal degeneration as a remote effect of cancer, generally small-cell undifferentiated cervical carcinoma, or oat cell carcinoma of the lung. This is an immunologically mediated retinopathy presumably caused by a cross-reactive antigenicity between certain carcinomas and the retina. Loss of vision and retinopathy may be rapid or slow. With severe loss of vision, the ERG will be severely abnormal, even in the presence of a normal fundus examination.

Thioridazine is a phenothiazine that has been demonstrated to cause severe retinal toxicity and a pigmentary retinopathy similar to that seen with RP or choroideremia. ERG testing may demonstrate subnormal a and b wave responses.

Chlorpromazine, when taken for long duration at a high dose, has also caused a pigmentary retinopathy. Retinal function is not significantly affected. The retinopathy may regress when the drug is discontinued.

Chloroquine, when taken for a prolonged duration at high dose, may also cause a pigmentary retinopathy. Unlike in RP, dark adaptometry may be normal, or just mildly abnormal. Bone-spicules may be seen in the mid and far periphery and a bulls-eye maculopathy may be noted.

Pigmented paravenous retinochoroidal atrophy has been reported in association with a family history of tuberculosis, syphilis, rubella, or in association with tuberculosis or meningoencephalitis. The pigment clumping is in association with the retinal veins and is generally stable over time. The ERG may be mildly to moderately abnormal, but the EOG can be severely abnormal.

A traumatic injury may lead to a unilateral pigmentary retinopathy simulating unilateral RP.

Diffuse unilateral subacute neuroretinitis is a panretinal pigmentary retinopathy resulting from an infection with various kinds of worms. The patient has normal vision until a certain age when a visual disturbance develops. The retina may appear normal or show evidence of early retinal degeneration. A living nematode is sometimes observed. The funduscopic picture may eventually resemble that seen in advanced RP. The fellow eye remains normal. The course is as expected for an acquired parasitic infection.

Retinal pigment hypertrophy, or grouped pigmentation of the retina, also known as "bear track pigmentation" is a benign and congenital condition. Areas of pigment hypertrophy are scattered throughout the retina. Retinal function tests are normal.

Stem Cells

Human mesenchymal stem cells (hMSCs) are able to differentiate into different tissues in vitro, are multipotent, and are capable of renewing themselves. However, a major difference between the in vivo hMSCs and the manufactured pharmaceutical product is that in vivo hMSCs also provide trophic factors which induce intrinsic stem cells to repair tissue and to modulate the immune system.

The original premise was that stem cells would migrate to the site of injury and stimulate tissue repair. It now appears that the original theory was incorrect. hMSCs have been determined to be perivascular cells. They express cellular markers CD10, CD13, CD44, CD73, CD90, CD105, and CD146. hMSCs do not differentiate into the damaged tissue, but provide the signaling immunomodulatory and trophic factors that stimulate other tissue-specific progenitor cells to regenerate the injured tissue. Rather than the term "stem cells," the new proposed term is "Medicinal Signaling Cells." hMSCs have high immunomodulatory potential. They alter antigen-presenting maturation, inhibit T-cell expansion and recognition, and promote lymphocyte T helper (Th2) response by increasing interleukin 10 (IL-10) and inhibiting tumor necrosis factor-alpha (TNF-α) and interferon-gamma (IFN-γ).

There are two main types of mesenchymal stem cells (MSCs) used in clinical studies. Adult MSCs include those derived from bone marrow, peripheral blood, adipose tissue, and dental pulp and neonatal-derived MSCs from umbilical cord, amnion, and placenta. Bone-marrow-derived MSCs are the most popularly used cells in clinical trials and have been shown to be beneficial in clinically relevant models.

Induced pluripotent stem cells or iPSC are pluripotent stem cells that can be derived from a somatic cell, such as skin or blood cells. In 2006, Yamanaka and

Takahashi demonstrated that the introduction of four specific genes could change somatic into pluripotent cells. As such, they bypass the ethical dilemma of destroying an embryo to produce embryonic stem cells. Like embryonic stem cells, there is the risk of tumor formation. In addition, the efficiency of reprogramming a somatic cell to an iPS cell is low.

Chapter 2
Treatments for Retinitis Pigmentosa

From an historical perspective, it was once thought that limited light exposure might slow the progression of retinitis pigmentosa (RP), but no effect was found. Likewise, there was no benefit of an increased intake of vitamin A, although vitamin E intake was found to be deleterious.

Gene-independent, neuroprotective strategies are under study, including: rod-derived cone viability factor, N-acetyl cysteine, and NFE2-like bZIP transcription factor 2 (previously known as *NRF2*). Gene-specific therapies are progressing, along with strategies for end-stage disease in which there are no rods or cones (e.g., optogenetics).

At the present time, the only FDA approved treatment is Luxturna® (voretigene neparvovec) for a small sub-population of patients that have the RPE65 mutation, which represents 0.3–1% of total RP cases. Luxturna is an adeno-associated virus vector-based gene therapy.

Twelve patients (mean age 13.5 years ±7.9 years) were treated with Luxturna with 1 year of follow-up. They reported an improvement in best corrected visual acuity (BCVA) of −0.21 (±0.14; $P < 0.001$) an improvement on a full-field stimulus threshold (FST) test white light sensitivity thresholds of −26.3 (±10.7, $P < 0.001$), and using chromatic pupillometry, an improvement in maximum pupillary constriction in response to blue and white stimulus at 10 lux level ($P < 0.05$). There was an enlargement of the semi-automated kinetic visual field (SKVF) using I4e ($1921.7 \pm 3247.3^{\circ 2}$; $P = 0.011$) and III4e ($2478 \pm 3659.7^{\circ 2}$; $P < 0.001$).

Bilateral retinal atrophy was observed in 4/12 patients at 6 months of follow-up, but this adverse event was not associated with worse outcomes on the efficacy measures, except in the SKVF using I4e stimulus size, in which patients with retinal atrophy showed significantly less improvement in their eyes ($159.9 \pm 1309.9^{\circ}$) compared to the eyes of patients who were not experiencing retinal atrophy ($2802.6 \pm 3589.6^{\circ}$; $P = 0.033$).

Luxturna costs $425,000 per eye, for one treatment.

J. N. Weiss, *Clinical Trials in Retinitis Pigmentosa Treatment*,
https://doi.org/10.1007/978-3-031-58799-3_2

However, Oxford Eye Hospital reported a retrospective study of 5 Luxturna treated patients which did not find significant improvement in BCVA. The BCVA for treated patients (19–51 years, mean 35.6) was similar at the last follow-up (1.17 LogMAR; ±0.38) to the mean BCVA at baseline (1.15 LogMAR; ±0.47; $P = 0.93$). Improvements were observed in FST testing.

Ghent University Hospital reported that a study of eight treated Belgian patients (6–54 years, mean 27.5) did not demonstrate a statistically significant improvement in BCVA, but an improvement in FST testing was noted.

A potential treatment for RP is the use of optogenetics to control neuron activity with light. Genes for light sensitive proteins are introduced into cells, so they may be controlled using light. Spatial selectivity is important, that is, there needs to be a spectral separation, where channels are activated by different wavelengths of light.

The RESTORE clinical trial, conducted by Nanoscope Therapeutics Inc., is a Phase 2b multicenter, randomized, double-masked, sham-controlled clinical trial (clinical trials NCT04945772) of their product, multi-characteristic opsin (MCO)-010 (sonpiretigene isteparvovec), and an ambient-light activatable MCO optogenetic therapy. Eighteen patients with severe vision impairment due to RP received a single intravitreal injection of MCO-010, and nine received a sham intravitreal injection.

Twelve-month results:

- 18 of 18 (100%) MCO 010 treated patients showed vision improvement in the multi-luminance Y-mobility test (MLYMT), multi-luminance shape discrimination test (MLSDT) or BCVA compared to 5 of 9 (55.6%) receiving placebo ($P = 0.007$).
- 17 of 18 (94.4%) MCO-010-treated patients showed vision improvement in the MLYMT or BCVA compared to 4 of 9 (44.4%) receiving placebo ($P = 0.008$).
- 16 of 18 (88.9%) MCO-010-treated patients demonstrated a 2 or more luminance-level improvement in the MLYMT or MLSDT compared to 4 of 9 (44.4%) receiving placebo ($P = 0.02$).
- 14 of 18 (77.8%) MCO-010-treated patients showed vision improvement in the MLSDT or BCVA compared to 3 of 9 (33.3%) receiving placebo ($P = 0.04$).

The most common ocular treatment emergent adverse events reported across treatment arms were anterior chamber cells, ocular hypertension, and conjunctival hemorrhage.

Chapter 3
Notes

The rationale for proprietary stem cell products has been to replace the damaged retinal tissue. However, this basic premise may be incorrect if the new cells do not engraft, but purely serve to stimulate other already present cells to heal. In addition, when the proprietary cells alone are injected, in the absence of the platelet-rich plasma, as occurs when autologous bone-marrow-derived stem cells (BMDsc) are used, there is an absence of the other beneficial growth factors.

Could this be the reason why no proprietary product used in retinal or optic nerve "stem cell" trials have proven more successful than the autologous bone marrow we use in the stem cell ophthalmology study (SCOTS)?

I am the Principal Investigator of the SCOTS I and II studies. SCOTS I began in 2012 and continues to the present time as SCOTS 2 (ClinicalTrials.gov ID NCT03011541). The original SCOTS1 had three arms. Arm 1 is the retrobulbar, subtenon, and intravenous injections of the autologous BMDsc, Arm 2 is the intravitreal and intravenous injections of BMDsc, and Arm 3 is the placement of the BMDsc in the subretinal space for retinal conditions, or directly into the optic nerve, for optic nerve conditions.

Arm 3 was discontinued in mid-2017, as in the absence of an anchor or scaffold, subretinal cell placement dissipates over time. Figures 3.1, 3.2, and 3.3 the visual results were similar to Arm 2. Arm 2 was discontinued later that same year, as the results were similar to those obtained in Arm 1. We have been exclusively been performing Arm I since that time.

Retinal detachment has been a significant complication of the subretinal placement of cells. Cells migrate to the point of instrument insertion and produce membranes, opening the hole in the retina and producing a retinal detachment. I developed a shelved, self-sealing needle and there have been no retinal detachments when I was still performing Arm 3 of SCOTS. No laser or gas was needed after cell insertion.

However, is direct placement of cells even necessary? As you can see, the majority of cells disappear over time. Sometimes, pigment remains (see below) (Fig. 3.4).

J. N. Weiss, *Clinical Trials in Retinitis Pigmentosa Treatment*,
https://doi.org/10.1007/978-3-031-58799-3_3

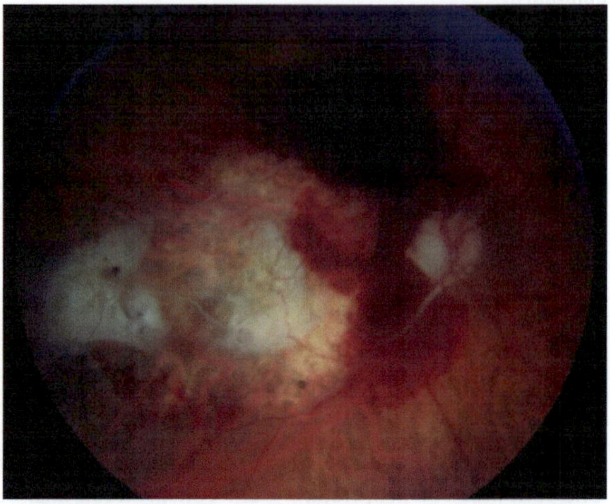

Fig. 3.1 One-week postoperative subretinal cell placement. At the time of surgery, the entire area of atrophy was covered with cells. Despite instructions to the contrary, the patient reported sleeping on their right side. Note that the cells have migrated to the right

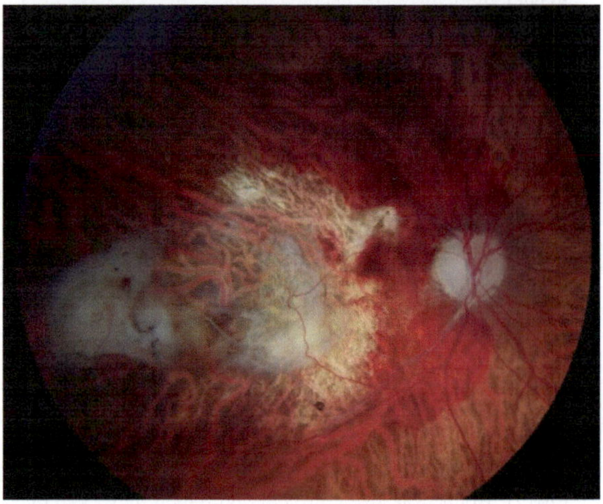

Fig. 3.2 Three weeks postoperatively. The cells continue to dissipate

In addition, what is the rationale for intravitreal injections? If there is no engraftment, but a stimulation of already present cells, might subtenon and retrobulbar injections work equally as well? That is what we found in SCOTS. Sometimes, what seems the most obvious, isn't.

Years ago, I was an investigator in the early treatment diabetes retinopathy study. The diabetic retinopathy study proved that laser photocoagulation in the presence of significant proliferative diabetic retinopathy, as defined in the study, was effective in reducing blindness. It seemed obvious that earlier treatment would result in better results. And yet it didn't. That's why I say what seems "obvious" isn't always, which is why we do studies, and not just accept a theory without proof. Hypothesis must fit facts, not the other way around.

As the injected cells are opaque, patients who received an intravitreal injection in Arm 2 of SCOTS complained of seeing a "glob" or a "cloud" in their vision. In a

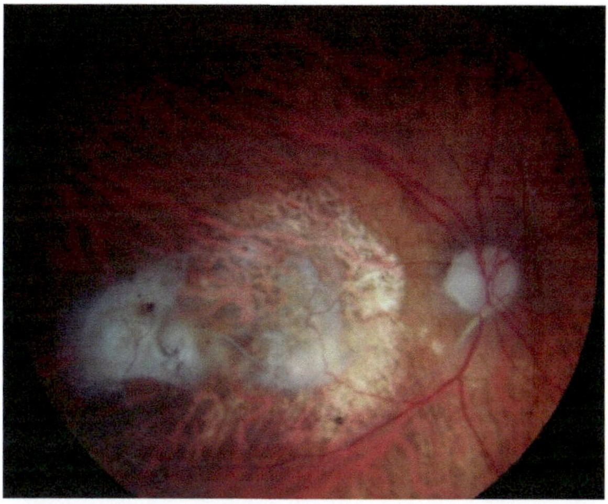

Fig. 3.3 Ten weeks postoperatively. The surgically implanted cells have disappeared

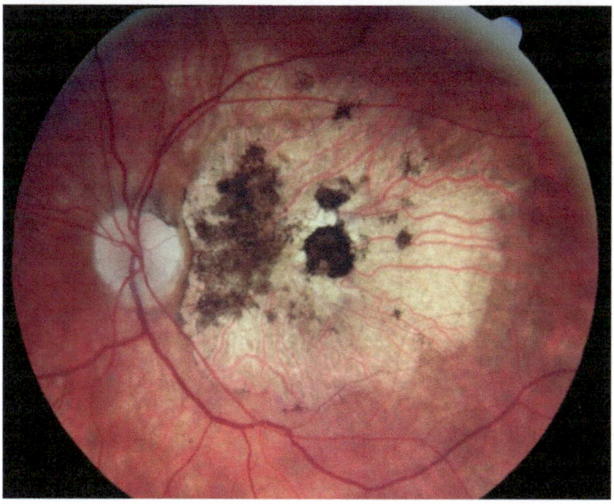

Fig. 3.4 Five months postoperatively

vitrectomized eye, the cells dissipated with a more severe decrease in the patient's vision after the procedure. However, we found that the visual results of the intravitreal injection were similar to those undergoing the retrobulbar and subtenon injections. As a result, we no longer perform intravitreal injections. Patients are happy and there is a lower potential risk of a complication.

Part I
Stem Cell Studies

Chapter 4
Completed Stem Cell Studies

Completed Studies

United States

Safety of Repeat Intravitreal Injection of Human Retinal Progenitor Cells (jCell) in Adult Subjects with Retinitis Pigmentosa

ClinicalTrials.gov ID NCT04604899

Sponsor jCyte, Inc
Information provided by jCyte, Inc (Responsible Party)
Last Update Posted 2022-08-10

Brief Summary
The primary objective of the study is to assess the safety of repeat injection of human retinal progenitor cells (jCell) in adult subjects with retinitis pigmentosa (RP) that have previously been treated with jCell.

Detailed Description
This is a prospective, multi-center, single arm, Phase 2 study of human retinal progenitor cells (jCell) for the treatment of RP. The study will include only subjects previously treated with jCell.

To assess reinjection of a previously treated eye, subjects who have previously been treated with jCell and desire a second treatment in the same eye will be enrolled. Subjects must have completed at least 12 months of follow-up since the prior injection of jCell. Subjects who have had both eyes previously treated with jCell will only have one eye retreated; the eye to be retreated will preferably be the better seeing eye, but exceptions may be made by the study investigator, taking into consideration best corrected visual acuity (BCVA), prior response to treatment, and

J. N. Weiss, *Clinical Trials in Retinitis Pigmentosa Treatment*,
https://doi.org/10.1007/978-3-031-58799-3_4

any other medical conditions that may indicate which eye is the best candidate for retreatment. Subjects will be followed for 12 months for safety and efficacy.

Official Title

A Phase 2 Study of the Safety of Repeat Intravitreal Injection of Human Retinal Progenitor Cells (jCell) in Adult Subjects with Retinitis Pigmentosa (RP)

Conditions

Retinitis Pigmentosa

Intervention/Treatment

Biological: human retinal progenitor cells
Interventional Model: Single Group Assignment
Masking: None (Open Label)

Arms and interventions

Participant group/arm	Intervention/treatment
Experimental: Retreated subjects Subjects receiving human retinal progenitor cells (jCell) who have previously received jCell is a jCyte study	Biological: human retinal progenitor cells • Single intravitreal injection of 6.0 million human retinal progenitor cells (hRPC) • Other Names: – jCell

Primary outcome measures

Outcome measure	Measure description	Time frame
Safety of intravitreal injection of hRPC	Assessed by proportion of subjects with treatment emergent adverse events	12 months

Secondary outcome measures

Outcome measure	Measure description	Time frame
Best corrected visual acuity	Assessed by E-ETDRS	12 months
Visual fields	The Octopus 900 will be used for kinetic visual field testing using a specified target of V4e for more severe subjects and a target of III4e and V4e for better seeing subjects	12 months
Contrast sensitivity	The Beethoven System will be used to capture the peak mean contrast sensitivity threshold value at any given spatial frequency	12 months
Mobility	Maze testing	12 months

Results

Arm/Group Title	Retreated Subjects
Arm/Group Description	Subjects receiving human retinal progenitor cells (jCell) who have previously received jCell is a jCyte study Human retinal progenitor cells: single intravitreal injection of 6.0 million human retinal progenitor cells (hRPC)
Quality Control Review Comment provided by the National Library of Medicine: 1. The Enrollment number appears inconsistent with information in other parts of the record	

Period Title: Overall Study	
Started	30[a]
Completed	23
Not Completed	7

[a] 31 total subjects were enrolled but only 30 were treated; one was determined to have met the exclusion criteria after enrollment but prior to treatment

1. Primary Outcome:	
Title	Safety of Intravitreal Injection of hRPC
Description	Assessed by proportion of subjects with treatment emergent adverse events (TEAE)
Time Frame	12 months
Outcome Measure Data	
Analysis Population Description	
Safety population: all subjects who receive any study treatment	
Overall Number of Participants Analyzed	30
Measure Type: Number Unit of Measure: Subjects	
Subjects with any TEAEs	15 50%
Subjects with any TEAEs related/ possibly related to study drug	6 20%
Subjects with any serious TEAEs	6 20%
Subjects with any serious TEAEs related/possibly related to study drug	2 6.7%
Subjects with any severe TEAEs related/possibly related to study drug	1 3.3%
2. Secondary Outcome:	
Title	Best Corrected Visual Acuity
Description	Assessed by E-ETDRS
Time Frame	12 months
Outcome Measure Data Not Reported	
3. Secondary Outcome:	
Title	Visual Fields
Description	The Octopus 900 will be used for kinetic visual field testing using a specified target of V4e for more severe subjects and a target of III4e and V4e for better seeing subjects
Time Frame	12 months
Outcome Measure Data Not Reported	
4. Secondary Outcome:	
Title	Contrast Sensitivity
Description	The Beethoven System will be used to capture the peak mean contrast sensitivity threshold value at any given spatial frequency
Time Frame	12 months

Outcome Measure Data Not Reported	
5. Secondary Outcome:	
Title	Mobility
Description	Maze testing
Time Frame	12 months
Outcome Measure Data Not Reported	
▼ Adverse Events	
Time Frame	12 months
Adverse Event Reporting Description	[Not specified]
All-Cause Mortality	
	Retreated Subjects
	Affected/At Risk (%)
Total	2/30 (6.67%)
Serious Adverse Events	
	Retreated Subjects
	Affected/At Risk (%)
Total	6/30 (20%)
Cardiac disorders	
Acute left ventricular failure[a]	1/30 (3.33%)
Ear and labyrinth disorders	
Vertigo positional[a]	1/30 (3.33%)
Eye disorders	
Tractional retinal detachment[a]	1/30 (3.33%)
Vitreoretinal traction syndrome[a]	1/30 (3.33%)
Infections and infestations	
COVID-19[a]	1/30 (3.33%)
COVID-19 pneumonia[a]	1/30 (3.33%)
Pneumonia[a]	1/30 (3.33%)
Neoplasms benign, malignant and unspecified (incl cysts and polyps)	
Non-small cell lung cancer[a]	1/30 (3.33%)
Nervous system disorders	
Cerebrovascular accident[a]	1/30 (3.33%)
Psychiatric disorders	
Hallucination[a]	1/30 (3.33%)
Respiratory, thoracic and mediastinal disorders	
Chronic obstructive pulmonary disease[a]	1/30 (3.33%)
Pleural effusion[a]	1/30 (3.33%)
Pulmonary embolism[a]	1/30 (3.33%)
Quality Control Review Comment provided by the National Library of Medicine: 1. Required information appears to be missing	
Other (Not Including Serious) Adverse Events	
Frequency Threshold for Reporting Other Adverse Events	5%
	Retreated Subjects
	Affected/At Risk (%)

Total	8/30 (26.67%)
Eye disorders	
Conjunctival hemorrhage[a]	6/30 (20%)
Infections and infestations	
COVID-19[a]	2/30 (6.67%)
Quality Control Review Comment provided by the National Library of Medicine: 1. Required information appears to be missing	

[a] Indicates events were collected by systematic assessment

Completed

United States

Safety and Efficacy of Intravitreal Injection of Human Retinal Progenitor Cells in Adults with Retinitis Pigmentosa

ClinicalTrials.gov ID NCT03073733

Sponsor jCyte, Inc
Information provided by jCyte, Inc (Responsible Party)
Last Update Posted 2022-04-04

Brief Summary
This study evaluates the changes in visual function at 12 months following a single injection of human retinal progenitor cells compared to sham-treated controls in a cohort of adult subjects with RP.

Detailed Description
There is no effective treatment for RP; once photoreceptors are lost, they do not regenerate. The rate of deterioration of vision varies from person to person, with most people with RP legally blind by age 40. Preclinical studies demonstrated that transplantation of retinal progenitor cells into the eye can result in both photoreceptor replacement and significant slowing of host photoreceptor loss. Thus, the primary goal of this therapy is to preserve, and potentially improve, vision by intervening in the disease at a time when dystrophic host photoreceptors can be protected and reactivated. Based on the demonstration of acceptable safety and tolerability in a phase 1/2a study, this phase 2b study is designed as a controlled comparison of the changes in visual function and functional vision in subjects who receive a single jCell injection in comparison with a comparable sham-treated control group of subjects with RP.

Official Title
A Prospective, Multicenter, Randomized, Study of the Safety and Efficacy of Intravitreal Injection of Human Retinal Progenitor Cells (jCell) in Adult Subjects with Retinitis Pigmentosa (RP)

Conditions
Retinitis Pigmentosa

Study Type
Interventional

Enrollment (Actual)
84

Intervention/Treatment
Biological: human retinal progenitor cells
Other: Mock injection

Phase
Phase 2

Study Start (Actual)
2017-03-01

Primary Completion (Actual)
2020-11-13

Study Completion (Actual)
2020-11-13

Primary Purpose: Treatment
Allocation: Randomized
Interventional Model: Parallel Assignment
Masking: Double

Arms and interventions

Participant group/arm	Intervention/treatment
Experimental: Test (jCell injection) dose level 1 single intravitreal injection of 3.0 × 10e6 human retinal progenitor cells into the eye with the poorest visual acuity or, if vision is comparable in both eyes, the non-dominant eye	Biological: human retinal progenitor cells • Live suspension of 3.0 or 6.0 × 10e6 human retinal progenitor cells (hRPC) suspended in clinical grade medium injected intravitreally under local anesthesia • Other Names: – jCell
Other: Sham-treated Control a mock injection will be performed on the eye with the poorest vision in each Control subject (designated as the "study eye")	Other: Mock injection • Pressing the hub of a syringe with no needle against the eye to mimic intravitreal injection
Experimental: test (jCell injection) dose level 2 single intravitreal injection of 6.0 × 10e6 human retinal progenitor cells into the eye with the poorest visual acuity or, if vision is comparable in both eyes, the non-dominant eye	Biological: human retinal progenitor cells • Live suspension of 3.0 or 6.0 × 10e6 human retinal progenitor cells (hRPC) suspended in clinical grade medium injected intravitreally under local anesthesia • Other Names: – jCell

Primary outcome measures

Outcome measure	Measure description	Time frame
Best Corrected Visual Acuity (BCVA)	Mean change in BCVA in study eye from baseline to month 12 as assessed by E-ETDRS in ITT population. A letter score is used to compare change over time, with a higher number of letters representing better visual function, and a lower number of letters representing worse visual function. For example, 85 letters is equivalent to 20/20 visual acuity and 5 letters is equivalent to 20/800 visual acuity. A change value is derived for each subject by taking the letter score at 12 months and subtracting the letter score at baseline. A mean of all change values is then calculated for each arm	12 months

Secondary outcome measures

Outcome measure	Measure description	Time frame
Contrast Sensitivity (CS) at 1.0 CPD	Assessment of the ability to detect changes in shades of grey, as measured with a vertical striped pattern that varies in width (cycles per degree or CPD); CS thresholds are created by taking the mean of multiple trials at each pattern width. A CS curve is created using a minimum of three pattern widths, one at the subject's peak or highest sensitivity, and then one larger and smaller pattern width on either side of the peak. For example, if a subject's CS peak appears to be at 2.0 CPD, then additional testing occurs at 1.0 and 4.0 CPD. RP patients have suppressed CS curves and the most common pattern widths are at 0.5, 1.0, 2.0, and 4.0 CPD. Severely impaired subjects (e.g., BCVA <20/400) usually have flat curves with low values (e.g., 1.28), while in mildly impaired RP subjects the values can be higher (e.g., 7.12), but are rarely near normal. These data represent mean change in CS from baseline to 12 months, with greater values representing greater improvement in visual function	12 months
Kinetic Visual Field (KVF)	Mean change in total area (degrees squared) of all islands of vision from baseline to 12 months	12 months
Low Luminance Mobility Test (LLMT)	The LLMT identifies the performance of RP patients as they walk along an indoor pathway of arrows and obstacles at varying lighting levels. The Critical Illumination Level (CIL) is the light level below which the patient has a markedly slower pace and more errors than all light levels above (brighter than) that point. The LLMT uses light levels that go from very dim (0.12 lux) to a bright indoor room (500 lux), with evenly spaced increments that increase light by doubling the brightness of the room from the prior level. These evenly spaced light levels have been converted to a scale score to enable easier calculation of change scores. The dimmest light level of 0 lux (completely dark room) corresponds to a scale score of 13, whereas the brightest light level of 500 lux corresponds to a scale score of 0. A positive scale score change from baseline to 12 months represents improvement in low light vision, whereas a negative scale score change represents a decline in low light vision	12 months

Low Vision Functional Questionnaire (Visual Ability)	The VA LV VFQ-48 (VFQ) is used to capture changes in patients' self-reporting of their difficulty with reading, mobility and performing other daily living activities affected by visual impairment. There are 4 scales on the VFQ including Visual Information, Reading, Visual Motor, and Mobility. A fifth value, Visual Ability, is an aggregate score of the 4 scales, measured in units called logits, and is calculated for each person based on item weighting using Rasch analysis. Visual Ability is used broadly to represent changes in subject-reported outcomes from visit to visit. Higher positive values on the Visual Ability score represent better function and less impairment, whereas lower or negatives scores represent worse function or more impairment. Change in the Visual Ability scale on the VFQ is calculated by taking a subject's score at 12 months and subtracting from it the baseline score	12 months
Safety of Intravitreal Injection of Retinal Progenitor Cells (RPC)	Assessed by treatment emergent adverse events, immunogenicity and safety visual assessments	12 months

General Publications

No publications available

Results

Recruitment Details

85 subjects were enrolled; 84 subjects were randomized

Pre-assignment Details

One subject received a 4.0 × 10e6 dose prior to a major protocol amendment that excluded this dose group; this subject is not included in the analyses presented.

Outcome Measures

1. Best Corrected Visual Acuity (BCVA)

Type: Primary | Time Frame: 12 months

Arm/group title	Sham-treated control	Test (jCell injection) dose level 1	Test (jCell injection) dose level 2
Arm/Group Description	Mock injection: pressing the hub of a syringe with no needle against the study eye to mimic intravitreal injection	Single intravitreal injection of 3.0 × 10e6 retinal progenitor cells into the study eye	Single intravitreal injection of 6.0 × 10e6 retinal progenitor cells into the study eye
Started	29	27	27
Completed	28	26	26
Not Completed	1	1	1
Reason Not Completed			

Lost to Follow-up	1	0	0
Physician Decision	0	1	0
Withdrawal by Subject	0	0	1

Description	Mean change in BCVA in study eye from baseline to month 12 as assessed by E-ETDRS in ITT population. A letter score is used to compare change over time, with a higher number of letters representing better visual function, and a lower number of letters representing worse visual function. For example, 85 letters are equivalent to 20/20 visual acuity and 5 letters are equivalent to 20/800 visual acuity. A change value is derived for each subject by taking the letter score at 12 months and subtracting the letter score at baseline. A mean of all change values is then calculated for each arm
Time Frame	12 months
Analysis Population Description	ITT: All randomized subjects who provide any post-randomization data. One subject received a 4.0 × 10e6 dose prior to a protocol amendment that excluded this dose level; this subject is not included in these analyses. In addition, of the 83 remaining subjects to be enrolled and randomized, 80 completed the study

Overall Number of Participants Analyzed	28	26	26
Mean (Standard Deviation) | Unit of Measure: Letters correct	3.9(9.92)	1.3(14.14)	2.6(21.53)

Sham-treated control	Test (jCell injection) dose level 1	Test (jCell injection) dose level 2	Total
Mock injection: pressing the hub of a syringe with no needle against the study eye to mimic intravitreal injection	Single intravitreal injection of 3.0 × 10e6 retinal progenitor cells into the study eye	Single intravitreal injection of 6.0 × 10e6 retinal progenitor cells into the study eye	Total of all reporting groups
29	27	27	83
29 participants	27 participants	27 participants	83 participants
517.2%	414.8%	725.9%	1619.3%
2482.8%	2385.2%	2074.1%	6780.7%
00.0%	00.0%	00.0%	00.0%
29 participants	27 participants	27 participants	83 participants
29 participants	27 participants	27 participants	83 participants
1241.4%	1244.4%	1451.9%	3845.8%
1758.6%	1555.6%	1348.1%	4554.2%

Outcome measures

Arm/group title	Sham-treated control	Test (jCell injection) dose level 1	Test (jCell injection) dose level 2
Arm/Group Description	Mock injection: pressing the hub of a syringe with no needle against the study eye to mimic intravitreal injection	Single intravitreal injection of 3.0 × 10e6 retinal progenitor cells into the study eye	Single intravitreal injection of 6.0 × 10e6 retinal progenitor cells into the study eye
Overall Number of Participants Analyzed	29	27	27
Subjects with TEAE[a]	15	20	21
Subjects with related/possibly related TEAE[a]	7	14	13
Subjects with severe TEAE[a]	0	3	1
Subjects with SAE[a]	0	1	0
Subjects with CME absent at baseline and present at M12 (OCT)[a]	1	0	0
Subjects with clinically significant abnormal conjunctiva absent at baseline and present at M12[a]	0	2	0
Subjects with clinically significant abnormal sclera absent at baseline and present at M12[a]	0	1	0
Subjects with clinically significant abnormal AC flare absent at baseline and present at M12[a]	0	0	0

[a] Measure Type: Number I Unit of Measure: participants

Completed

United States

Safety of a Single, Intravitreal Injection of Human Retinal Progenitor Cells (jCell) in Retinitis Pigmentosa

ClinicalTrials.gov ID NCT02320812

Sponsor jCyte, Inc
Information provided by jCyte, Inc (Responsible Party)
Last Update Posted 2019-03-05

Brief Summary
This study evaluates the safety and potential activity of a single dose of live human retinal progenitor cells (jCell) administered to adults with RP. Four different dose levels of cells will be assessed in each of two groups of patients.

Detailed Description
The primary purpose of this study is to test the safety and tolerability of the administration of a single dose of jCell to adults with RP.

The goal of jCell therapy is to preserve vision by intervening in the disease at a time when host photoreceptors can be protected and potentially reactivated.

Human allogeneic retinal progenitor cells will be injected into adults with advanced RP to see if the procedure is safe, if the cells survive, and whether they have any impact on the visual status of the patients.

Conditions
Retinitis Pigmentosa (RP)

Study Type
Interventional

Enrollment (Actual)
28

Intervention/Treatment
Biological: human retinal progenitor cells

Phase
Phase 1 Phase 2

Study Start
2015-06

Primary Completion (Actual)
2017-07-19

Study Completion (Actual)
2017 07-19

Interventional Model: Single Group Assignment
Masking: None (Open Label)

Arms and interventions

Participant group/arm	Intervention/treatment
Experimental: Treated subjects human retinal progenitor cells	Biological: human retinal progenitor cells • Single intravitreal injection of 0.5–3.0 million human retinal progenitor cells (hRPC) • Other Names: – jCell

Primary outcome measures

Outcome measure	Measure description	Time frame
Number of Subjects With Adverse Events as a Measure of Safety and Tolerability	Proportion of subjects with treatment emergent adverse events (TEAE), related TEAE and severe TEAE	12 months

Secondary outcome measures

Outcome measure	Measure description	Time frame
Change in Mean Best Corrected Visual Acuity (BCVA)	Change in mean best corrected visual acuity in test eye versus untreated eye; BCVA is measured using an eye chart and is reported as the number of letters read correctly (ranging from 0 to 100 letters) in the study eye. The lower the number of letters read correctly on the eye chart, the worse the vision (or visual acuity). A positive change from baseline indicates an improvement and a negative change from baseline indicates a worsening. Change between baseline and month 12 is reported	12 months

Results

Publications About Study Results

No publications available

Recruitment Details

85 subjects were enrolled; 84 subjects were randomized

Pre-assignment Details

One subject received a 4.0 × 10e6 dose prior to a major protocol amendment that excluded this dose group; this subject is not included in the analyses presented.

Arm/group title	Sham-treated control	Test (jCell injection) dose level 1	Test (jCell injection) dose level 2
Arm/Group Description	Mock injection: pressing the hub of a syringe with no needle against the study eye to mimic intravitreal injection	Single intravitreal injection of 3.0 × 10e6 retinal progenitor cells into the study eye	Single intravitreal injection of 6.0 × 10e6 retinal progenitor cells into the study eye
Started	29	27	27
Completed	28	26	26
Not Completed	1	1	1
Reason Not Completed			
Lost to Follow-up	1	0	0
Physician Decision	0	1	0
Withdrawal by Subject	0	0	1

Time Frame

One year

Adverse event reporting description

Sham-Treated Control	Test (jCell Injection) Dose Level 1	Test (jCell Injection) Dose Level 2
Mock injection: pressing the hub of a syringe with no needle against the study eye	Single intravitreal injection of 3.0 × 10e6 retinal progenitor cells into the study eye	Single intravitreal injection of 6.0 × 10e6 retinal progenitor cells into the study eye

Sham-Treated Control	Test (jCell Injection) Dose Level 1	Test (jCell Injection) Dose Level 2
Affected/at Risk (%)	Affected/at Risk (%)	Affected/at Risk (%)
0/29 (0.00%)	0/27 (0.00%)	0/27 (0.00%)

Sham-Treated Control		Test (jCell Injection) Dose Level 1		Test (jCell Injection) Dose Level 2	
Affected/at Risk (%)	# Events	Affected/at Risk (%)	# Events	Affected/at Risk (%)	# Events
0/29 (0.00%)		1/27 (3.70%)		0/27 (0.00%)	
0/29 (0.00%)	0	1/27 (3.70%)	1	0/27 (0.00%)	0

Sham-Treated Control		Test (jCell Injection) Dose Level 1		Test (jCell Injection) Dose Level 2	
Affected/at Risk (%)	# Events	Affected/at Risk (%)	# Events	Affected/at Risk (%)	# Events
13/29 (44.83%)		18/27 (66.67%)		14/27 (51.85%)	
0/29 (0.00%)	0	0/27 (0.00%)	0	3/27 (11.11%)	3
0/29 (0.00%)	0	2/27 (7.41%)	2	0/27 (0.00%)	0
5/29 (17.24%)	5	9/27 (33.33%)	9	6/27 (22.22%)	6
1/29 (3.45%)	1	2/27 (7.41%)	3	0/27 (0.00%)	0
0/29 (0.00%)	0	1/27 (3.70%)	1	2/27 (7.41%)	2
0/29 (0.00%)	0	5/27 (18.52%)	6	1/27 (3.70%)	1
3/29 (10.34%)	3	4/27 (14.81%)	4	3/27 (11.11%)	3
2/29 (6.90%)	2	0/27 (0.00%)	0	0/27 (0.00%)	0
2/29 (6.90%)	2	0/27 (0.00%)	0	0/27 (0.00%)	0
1/29 (3.45%)	1	1/27 (3.70%)	1	2/27 (7.41%)	2
0/29 (0.00%)	0	2/27 (7.41%)	2	0/27 (0.00%)	0
0/29 (0.00%)	0	2/27 (7.41%)	2	1/27 (3.70%)	1
1/29 (3.45%)	1	4/27 (14.81%)	4	1/27 (3.70%)	1
0/29 (0.00%)	0	2/27 (7.41%)	2	0/27 (0.00%)	0

Discussion

jCell (famzeretcel, jCyte) is an allogeneic retinal progenitor cell product. Immunosuppressive therapy is not required for treatment. Positive results are reported in a subset of patients of with better baseline visual acuity (20/80 to 20/800).

Eighty-three patients were randomly assigned to two active treatment groups and a sham treatment group. The investigators tested two dosages (6.0 million cells and

3.0 million cells) in 27 patients each. Only the eye with worse vision was treated. There were 29 control patients. The primary end point was the mean change in BCVA from baseline to 12 months.

The investigators found that the treatment was well-tolerated though almost 50% of patients reported a treatment emergent adverse event (TEAE) considered related or possibly related to the treatment. 20% experienced a TEAE possibly related to the study drug. 20% of the TEAE were termed serious.

The 6.0 million (M) cell dose resulted in greater visual improvements compared to the 3.0M and sham groups. This dose achieved a mean improvement of 5.2 letters at 6 months and 4.6 letters at 12 months, but the differences did not reach significance. The 3.0M dose results were similar to those of the sham group.

The study utilized other testing in addition to visual acuity. The 6M dose at 12 months demonstrated a 90% increase in peak contrast sensitivity, a 132% improvement in kinetic visual field area, a 0.52-logit increase in the mobility-related visual function, and a 0.37-logit improvement in the overall visual ability, the last 2 of which were evaluated using the Visual Function Questionnaire-48.

More reliable endpoint measurements of BCVA were seen in patients with a 15-letter or less disparity between the eyes at baseline. Selecting out this patient group allowed statistical significance. There was a mean improvement in the 6.0M group compared with sham of 8.9 letters at 6 months ($p = 0.014$) and 9.4 letters at 12 months ($p = 0.019$). The secondary outcomes for the 6.0M group at 12 months also improved as a result: the mean increase in peak contrast sensitivity was 146%, kinetic visual field area 192%, mobility-related visual function 0.53 logit, and overall visual ability 0.42 logit.

A further subgroup analysis of patients with visual fields greater than 20° demonstrated better results. The BCVA change from baseline at 12 months in this group was 15.6 letters above Sham ($p = 0.029$).

One wonders whether the perforation of the sclera in the performance of an intravitreal injection, and the injection of a stimulating substance, is the actual cause of visual improvement, and not the actual "stem cells," as greater intraocular inflammation was observed in the 6M group.

Completed

Brazil

Autologous Bone-Marrow-Derived Stem Cells Transplantation for Retinitis Pigmentosa (RETICELL)

ClinicalTrials.gov ID NCT01560715

Sponsor University of Sao Paulo
Information provided by Rubens Camargo Siqueira, University of Sao Paulo (Responsible Party)
Last Update Posted 2017-07-21

Brief Summary
The purpose of this study is to evaluate the short-term safety and efficacy of a single intravitreal injection of autologous bone-marrow stem cells in patients with RP.

Detailed Description
A prospective phase II, nonrandomized open-label study of RP patients with best corrected ETDRS visual acuity (BCVA) worse than 20/200. Standardized ophthalmic evaluation will be perform at baseline and at weeks 1, 4, 12 and 24 (±1) following intravitreal injection of 10 × 10e6 bone-marrow stem cells/0.1 mL. Three measures will be used to evaluate the short-term safety of intravitreal of ABMDSC: (1) severe visual loss, defined as a drop in 15 letters on ETDRS visual acuity scale; (2) decrease in ERG response; and (3) decrease in $5^{\circ 2}$ on visual field; secondary safety outcomes: (1) increase in intra-ocular inflammation defined herein as anterior chamber cells and flare higher than 3+ for more than 1 month after injection according to a classification described elsewhere; (2) decrease in CMT more than 50 μm; (3)genesis of abnormal tissues (teratomas) or tumors; and (4) qualitative changes in retinal or choroidal perfusion, like macular c. Secondary outcome measures will be used to evaluate the short-term efficiency of intravitreal of ABMDSC: (1) improvement in ERG response; (2) increase in visual field: (3) increase in CSMT >50 μm and not related to macular edema; and (4) increase >5 letters on BCVA

Official Title
Phase 2 Study of Autologous Bone-Marrow-Derived Stem Cells Transplantation for Retinitis Pigmentosa

Conditions
Retinitis Pigmentosa

Study Type
Interventional

Enrollment (Actual)
50

Intervention/Treatment
Biological: intravitreal injection of autologous bone-marrow stem cells

Phase
Phase 2

Other Study ID Numbers
Rubens Siqueira

Study Start
2011-06

Primary Completion (Actual)
2013-01

Study Completion (Actual)
2013-06

Brazil
Locations

Sao Jose do Rio Preto, SP, Brazil, 15010-100
Centro de Pesquisa Rubens Siqueira

Eligibility Criteria
Ages Eligible for Study
18 Years to 75 Years (Adult, Older Adult)

Accepts Healthy Volunteer
No

Sexes Eligible for Study
All

Description

Inclusion Criteria
- Diagnosis of RP logarithm of minimum angle of resolution (logMAR) BCVA of 1.0 (Snellen equivalent, 20/200) or worse
- Visual Field less than 20°

Exclusion Criteria
- Previous ocular surgery other than cataract
- Presence of cataract or other media opacity that would influence ocular fundus documentation and adequate ERG and visual field evaluation
- Other ophthalmic diseases, such as glaucoma and uveitis
- Previous history of blood disorders, such as leukemia
- Known allergy to fluorescein or indocyanine green
- Known coagulation abnormalities or current use of anticoagulative medication other than aspirin.

Design Details
Primary Purpose: Treatment
Allocation: N/A
Interventional Model: Single Group Assignment
Masking: None (Open Label)

Arms and interventions

Participant group/arm	Intervention/treatment
Experimental: Experimental: Test group Retinitis pigmentosa patients with best corrected visual acuity (BCVA) worse than 20/200 or visual field less than 20°	Biological: intravitreal injection of autologous bone-marrow stem cells • One intravitreal injection of a 0.1-mL cell suspension containing around 10 × 10e6 bone-marrow mononuclear stem cells (BMMSC). All treatments were performed by a single retinal specialist using topical proparacaine drops under sterile conditions (eyelid speculum and povidone–iodine). Autologous BMMSC were injected into the vitreous cavity using a 27 gauge needle inserted through the inferotemporal pars plana 3.0–3.5 mm posterior to the limbus. After the injection, central retinal artery perfusion was confirmed with indirect ophthalmoscopy. Patients were instructed to instill one drop of 0.3% ciprofloxacin into the injected eye four times daily for 1 week after the procedure. • Other Names: – Autologous bone-marrow stem cells

Primary outcome measures

Outcome measure	Measure description	Time frame
ETDRS Visual acuity change		Day 1 to day 365

Sponsor
University of Sao Paulo

Collaborators
No information provided

Investigators
- Principal Investigator: Rubens C Siqueira, MD, PhD, Sao Paulo University

General Publications

- Siqueira RC, Messias A, Voltarelli JC, Scott IU, Jorge R. Intravitreal injection of autologous bone marrow-derived mononuclear cells for hereditary retinal dystrophy: a phase I trial. Retina. 2011 Jun;31(6):1207–14. https://doi.org/10.1097/IAE.0b013e3181f9c242.
- Siqueira RC, Messias A, Messias K, Arcieri RS, Ruiz MA, Souza NF, Martins LC, Jorge R. Quality of life in patients with retinitis pigmentosa submitted to intravitreal use of bone marrow-derived stem cells (Reticell-clinical trial). Stem Cell Res Ther. 2015 Mar 14;6(1):29. https://doi.org/10.1186/s13287-015-0020-6.
- Siqueira RC. Stem cell therapy in retinal diseases? Rev Bras Hematol Hemoter. 2012;34(3):222–6. https://doi.org/10.5581/1516-8484.20120054. No abstract available.
- Siqueira RC, Messias A, Voltarelli JC, Messias K, Arcieri RS, Jorge R. Resolution of macular oedema associated with retinitis pigmentosa after intravitreal use of autologous BM-derived hematopoietic stem cell transplantation. Bone Marrow Transplant. 2013 Apr;48(4):612–3. https://doi.org/10.1038/bmt.2012.185. Epub 2012 Sep 24. No abstract available.

No Results Posted

Discussion
The original SCOTS study had the intravitreal injection (Arm 2) of autologous bone-marrow-derived cells. An analysis of the visual results demonstrated that there was no significant difference in the final visual acuity when the cells were injected subtenon and retrobulbar (Arm 1) as compared to intravitreally (Arm 2). For this reason, Arm 2 was discontinued in favor of Arm 1.

The intravitreal injection of an opaque substance led to patient complaints, more so if the opacity covered a focal area of vision, i.e., in RP, or in a previously vitrectomized eye. While Arm 1 produces what looks like a subtenon "hemorrhage," the affect is cosmetic, not functional.

Completed

Brazil

Autologous Bone-Marrow-Derived Stem Cell Transplantation for Retinitis Pigmentosa

ClinicalTrials.gov ID NCT01068561

Sponsor University of Sao Paulo
Information provided by Rubens Camargo Siqueira, University of Sao Paulo (Responsible Party)
Last Update Posted 2011-09-20

Brief Summary
The purpose of this study is to evaluate the short-term safety of a single intravitreal injection of autologous bone-marrow stem cells in patients with RP.

Detailed Description
A prospective phase I, nonrandomized open-label study of RP patients with best corrected ETDRS visual acuity (BCVA) worse than 20/200. Standardized ophthalmic evaluation will be perform at baseline and at weeks 1, 4, 12, and 24 (±1) following intravitreal injection of 10 × 10e6 bone-marrow stem cells/0.1 mL. Three measures will be used to evaluate the short-term safety of intravitreal of ABMDSC: (1) severe visual loss, defined as a drop in 15 letters on ETDRS visual acuity scale; (2) decrease in ERG response; and (3) decrease in $5^{\circ 2}$ on visual field; secondary safety outcomes: (1) increase in intra-ocular inflammation defined herein as anterior chamber cells and flare higher than 3+ for more than 1 month after injection according to a classification described elsewhere; (2) decrease in CMT more than 50 μm; (3) genesis of abnormal tissues (teratomas) or tumors; and (4) qualitative changes in

retinal or choroidal perfusion, such as macular nonperfusion. Secondary outcome measures will be used to evaluate the short-term efficiency of intravitreal of ABMDSC: (1) improvement in ERG response; (2) increase in visual field; (3) increase in CSMT >50 μm and not related to macular edema; and (4) increase >5 letters on BCVA

Official Title

Phase 1 Study of Autologous Bone-Marrow-Derived Stem Cells Transplantation for Retinitis Pigmentosa

Conditions

Retinitis Pigmentosa

Study Type

Interventional

Enrollment (Actual)

5

Intervention/Treatment

Biological: intravitreal injection of autologous bone-marrow stem cells

Phase

Phase 1

Other Study ID Numbers

CPRS

Study Start

2009-05

Primary Completion (Actual)

2010-01

Study Completion (Actual)

2010-02

Brazil

São Jose do Rio Preto, SP, Brazil, 15010-100

Eligibility Criteria

Ages Eligible for Study

18 Years and older (Adult, Older Adult)

Accepts Healthy Volunteer

No

Sexes Eligible for Study

All

Description

Inclusion Criteria

- Diagnosis of RP
- Logarithm of minimum angle of resolution (logMAR) BCVA of 1.0 (Snellen equivalent, 20/200) or worse

Exclusion Criteria

- Previous ocular surgery other than cataract
- Presence of cataract or other media opacity that would influence ocular fundus documentation and adequate ERG and visual field evaluation
- Other ophthalmic diseases, such as glaucoma and uveitis
- Previous history of blood disorders, such as leukemia
- Known allergy to fluorescein or indocyanine green
- Known coagulation abnormalities or current use of anticoagulative medication other than aspirin.

Design Details

Primary Purpose: Treatment
Allocation: Non-Randomized
Interventional Model: Single Group Assignment
Masking: None (Open Label)

Arms and interventions

Participant group/arm	Intervention/treatment
Experimental: Test group open-label study of retinitis pigmentosa patients with best corrected visual acuity (BCVA) worse than 20/200	Biological: intravitreal injection of autologous bone-marrow stem cells • One intravitreal injection of a 0.1-mL cell suspension containing around 10 × 10e6 bone-marrow mononuclear stem cells (BMMSC). All treatments were performed by a single retinal specialist using topical proparacaine drops under sterile conditions (eyelid speculum and povidone-iodine). Autologous BMMSC were injected into the vitreous cavity using a 27 gauge needle inserted through the inferotemporal pars plana 3.0–3.5 mm posterior to the limbus. After the injection, central retinal artery perfusion was confirmed with indirect ophthalmoscopy. Patients were instructed to instill one drop of 0.3% ciprofloxacin into the injected eye four times daily for 1 week after the procedure. • Other Names: – Autologous bone-marrow mononuclear stem cells

Primary outcome measures

Outcome measure	Measure description	Time frame
severe visual loss, defined as a drop in 15 letters on ETDRS visual acuity scale		3–6 months

Sponsor

University of Sao Paulo

Collaborators

No information provided

Investigators
- Principal Investigator: Rubens C Siqueira, MD, PhD, Research Center Rubens Siqueira, Catanduva Medicine School and São Paulo University

General Publications
No publications available

No Results Posted

Completed

Turkey

Spheroidal Mesenchymal Stem Cells in Retinitis Pigmentosa

ClinicalTrials.gov ID NCT05712148

Sponsor Acibadem University
Information provided by Berna Özkan, Acibadem University (Responsible Party)
Last Update Posted 2023-02-03

Brief Summary
Purpose: This prospective clinical case series aimed to evaluate the effect of suprachoroidal implantation of mesenchymal stem cells (MSCs) in the form of spheroids as a stem cell therapy for RP patients with relatively good visual acuity.

Methods: 15 eyes of 15 patients with RP who received suprachoroidal implantation of MSCs in the form of spheroids were included. BCVA, 10-2 and 30-2 visual field examination and multifocal electroretinography (mfERG) recordings were recorded at baseline, postoperative first, third and sixth months during follow-up.

Detailed Description
A prospective clinical trial was conducted in patients with RP at the department of ophthalmology, Acibadem University, Medical school. The study was approved by the Review Board of Cell, Organ and Tissue Transplantation Department of Turkish Ministry of Health. The study was performed in accordance with the Declaration of Helsinki.

Patient Evaluation: Fifteen patients with clinical and genetic diagnoses of RP were included in the study. Patients underwent ophthalmic examination including BCVA, intraocular pressure, anterior segment examination and dilated fundus examination (with topical tropicamide %1 and phenylephrine 2.5%). Each eye underwent spectral domain OCT scanning with Cirrus 5000 HD-OCT Angioplex (Carl Zeiss Meditec, Dublin, CA, USA), fundus autofluorescence and fundus fluorescein angiography (Heidelberg Engineering, Germany). MD (mean deviation) and PSD (pattern standard deviation) parameters of 10-2 and 30-2 visual field (VF) testing strategies with a Humphrey Field Analyzer model 750I (Carl Zeiss Meditec,

Dublin, CA, USA) were obtained. The electrophysiological function was assessed with mfERG evaluation (Monpack 3, Metrovision, France) according to the International Society for Clinical Electrophysiology of Vision (ISCEV) guidelines. BCVA was converted to the logarithm of the minimal angle of resolution (logMAR) equivalent.

The patients were excluded from the study, if they had (1) coexisting ocular pathology that may affect visual acuity, visual field and retinal morphology such as glaucoma, uveitis, previous vitreoretinal surgery, (2) coexisting cataract that may affect mfERG, visual field and/or ocular imaging, (3) refractive error that may affect measurements higher than +6.00D, lower than −6.00D, (4) coexisting systemic diseases that may affect visual function such as diabetes, vasculitis, rheumatological diseases and chronic immunosuppressive use, (5) periocular injection of platelet-rich blood and transcorneal electrical stimulation in previous 6 months, and previous ocular surgery.

Electrophysiologic Testing: After 30 min of dark adaptation and pupil dilatation with the application of one drop of tropicamide 1% (Tropamid, Bilim İlaç, Turkey), phenylephrine 2.5% (Mydfrin, Alcon), and proparacaine hydrochloride 0.5% (Alcaine, Alcon), ERG jet electrodes were placed. Multifocal electroretinographies were recorded after pupil dilatation. The stimulated retinal area was subtended in an area of 60° × 55°; 61 hexagon stimulants were used with alternating black (5 cd/m^2) and white (100 cd/m^2) stimulants. The concentric rings were analyzed according to International Society for Clinical Electrophysiology of Vision standards. The amplitude and latencies of P1, N1, and N2 components were recorded for every ring. The mean signal amplitudes (MSAs) of multifocal electroretinography (mfERG) in the macula (central 0–2°) and the peripheral (2–5°, 5–10°, 10–15°, and >15°) signal amplitude changes were evaluated separately.

Spheroidal Stem Cell Preparation: First passage umbilical cord-derived MSC was obtained from Labcell Cellular Laboratory Center which provides GMP (good manufacturing practices) conditions.

Spheroid Production: The spheroid production continued in GMP condition. First passage umbilical cord-derived MSCs were used in the production of spheroids. 100,000 MSCs were suspended with 100 μL. Serum-free medium (MSC NutriStem® XF Medium, Sartorius) containing %1 ciprofloxacin (Polipharma). Each well of the low-attachment 96 well plate was seeded with 100,000 cells in 100 μL medium. The cells were incubated at 37 °C for 48 h. At the end of 48 h, all spheroids were collected with a micropipette and transferred into Ringer's lactate solution (Osel/Biofleks) containing 1% HSA (CSL Behring). Spheroids were washed three times with Ringer's lactate solution containing 1% HAS (CSL Behring). 50 spheroids were produced for one patient (50 spheroids containing 5 × 10e6 cells were produced). 5 of 50 spheroids were reserved for quality control analysis. The remaining 45 spheroid membranes were embedded in the matrix.

Matrix Production and Cell Embedding Culture: Matrix mixture containing 225 μL cryoprecipitate + 22.5 μL calcium (Adeka) + 2.5 μL transamine (Haver) was added to each well of the 96 well plates. When the matrix became semi-solid,

45 spheroids were embedded in the middle of the matrix and incubated at 37 °C for 45 min. The matrix, which became completely solid after 45 min, was removed with the help of a scalpel, transferred into Ringer's lactate solution (Osel/Biofleks) containing 1% HAS (CSL Behring), and transferred to the operating room in this solution.

Quality Control Analysis Microbiological blood culture, fungal, endotoxin analysis and purity (ciprofloxacin <0.1 μg/mL), efficiency (adipocyte and cartilage differentiation analysis) Cell Count/Viability and flow cytometric analysis (CD34 <%2, CD45 <%4, CD90 >%80, HLA-DR <%4, CD105 >%60, CD73 >%70) were studied from the reserved spheroids for quality control analyses.

Surgical Technique: Patients underwent surgery under general anesthesia. The inferotemporal quadrant was chosen as the surgical area. 6.0 silk was used as the anchoring suture near the limbus between 4 and 5 o'clock. Conjunctiva and tenon were opened as 6 mm long cut at 6 mm from limbus parallel to the limbus and the edges of the cut were advanced 3 mm posteriorly. Two 8.0 vicryl sutures were used as traction sutures at the anterior corners of the conjunctiva. The tenon was dissected over the sclera posteriorly. Then we performed a 7 × 7 scleral flap. Anterior margin of the scleral flap was created at 8 mm from the limbus, parallel to the limbus with 30° ophthalmic knife. Two other half-thickness side cuts were made to create a U-shaped flap that has its base parallel to the lateral rectus muscle. Then starting from the infero-anterior edge, a deep scleral flap was dissected with a crescent blade. During the dissection black choroidal reflex should be observed all around the surface of the flap bed. The fibrin plug carrying spheroidal stem cells was placed over the choroid that was seen under the thin sclera. It was covered by the scleral flap and the flap was sutured to its original position from its edges with a 7.0 vicryl suture. Tenon and conjunctiva were closed separately with an 8.0 vicryl suture.

Official Title

Suprachoroidal Spheroidal Mesenchymal Stem Cell Implantation in Retinitis Pigmentosa: Clinical Results of 6 Month Follow-up

Conditions

Retinitis Pigmentosa
Stem Cell Transplant

Study Type

Interventional

Enrollment (Actual)

15

Intervention/Treatment

Biological: Stem cell implantation

Phase

Phase 1 Phase 2

Other Study ID Numbers
56733164/203 E.3858

Study Start (Actual)
2019-10-11

Primary Completion (Actual)
2022-01-30

Study Completion (Actual)
2022-06-14

Istanbul, Turkey
Acıbadem University

Eligibility Criteria
Ages Eligible for Study
(Child, Adult, Older Adult)

Accepts Healthy Volunteer
No

Sexes Eligible for Study
All

Description

Inclusion Criteria
- Clinical and genetic diagnosis of Retinitis Pigmentosa

Exclusion Criteria
- Coexisting ocular pathology that may affect visual acuity, visual field and retinal morphology, such as glaucoma, uveitis, previous vitreoretinal surgery
- Coexisting cataract that may affect mfERG, visual field and/or ocular imaging
- Refractive error that may affect measurements higher than +6.00D, lower than −6.00D
- Coexisting systemic diseases that may affect visual function such as diabetes, vasculitis, rheumatological diseases and chronic immunosuppressive use
- Periocular injection of platelet-rich blood and transcorneal electrical stimulation in previous 6 months and previous ocular surgery

Design Details
Primary Purpose: Supportive Care
Allocation: N/A
Interventional Model: Single Group Assignment
Masking: None (Open Label)

Arms and interventions

Participant group/arm	Intervention/treatment
Experimental: Retinitis Pigmentosa patients Suprachoroidal mesenchymal stem cell implanted Retinitis pigmentosa patients	Biological: Stem cell implantation • Suprachoroidal mesenchymal spheroidal stem cell implantation

Primary outcome measures

Outcome measure	Measure description	Time frame
Change in visual acuity after stem cell implantation in Retinitis Pigmentosa	Pre-implantation and post-implantation BCVA was converted to the logarithm of the minimal angle of resolution (logMAR) equivalent	3 years
Change in microperimetric evaluation after stem cell implantation in Retinitis Pigmentosa	MD (mean deviation) and PSD (pattern standard deviation) parameters of 10-2 and 30-2 visual field (VF) testing strategies with a Humphrey Field Analyzer model 750I (Carl Zeiss Meditec, Dublin, CA, USA) were obtained	3 years
Change in electrophysiological testing after stem cell implantation in Retinitis Pigmentosa	The electrophysiological function was assessed with mfERG evaluation (Monpack 3, Metrovision, France) according to the International Society for Clinical Electrophysiology of Vision (ISCEV) guidelines. After 30 min of dark adaptation and pupil dilatation with the application of one drop of tropicamide 1% (Tropamid, Bilim ˙Ilaç, Turkey), phenylephrine 2.5% (Mydfrin, Alcon), and proparacaine hydrochloride 0.5% (Alcaine, Alcon), ERG jet electrodes were placed. Multifocal electroretinographies were recorded after pupil dilatation. The concentric rings were analyzed according to International Society for Clinical Electrophysiology of Vision standards. The amplitude and latencies of P1, N1, and N2 components were recorded for every ring. The mean signal amplitudes (MSAs) of multifocal electroretinography (mfERG) in the macula (central 0–2°) and the peripheral (2–5°, 5–10°, 10–15°, and >15°) signal amplitude changes were evaluated separately.	3 years

Sponsor

Acibadem University

Collaborators

No information provided

Investigators

- Principal Investigator: Berna Özkan, Professor, Acibadem University
- Study Chair: Ercüment Ovalı, Professor, Acıbadem LabCell Cellular Therapy Center

General Publications

No publications available

Results Overview

No Study Results Posted on ClinicalTrials.gov for this Study

Discussion

If the results obtained with umbilical cord derived stem cells are not inferior to those obtained with autologous bone-marrow-derived stem cells, then the entire procedure is simplified. No longer will the patient require a bone-marrow aspiration in the operating room, as is presently done. This can now be an office-based procedure making it easier and less expensive to perform.

Chapter 5
Active, Recruiting Stem Cell Studies

United States

Recruiting

Stem Cell Ophthalmology Treatment Study II (SCOTS2)

ClinicalTrials.gov ID NCT03011541

Sponsor MD Stem Cells
Information provided by MD Stem Cells (Responsible Party)
Last Update Posted 2023-06-06

Brief Summary
This study will evaluate the use of autologous bone-marrow-derived stem cells (BMSC) for the treatment of retinal and optic nerve damage or disease.

Detailed Description
Eyes with loss of vision from retinal or optic nerve conditions generally considered irreversible will be treated with a combination of injections of autologous BMSC isolated from the bone marrow using standard medical and surgical practices. Retinal conditions may include degenerative, ischemic, or physical damage (examples may include macular degeneration, hereditary retinal dystrophies such as retinitis pigmentosa (RP), Stargardt disease, non-perfusion retinopathies, and post retinal detachment). Optic Nerve conditions may include degenerative, ischemic, or physical damage (examples may include optic nerve damage from glaucoma, compression, ischemic optic neuropathy, and optic atrophy). Injections may include retrobulbar, subtenon, intravitreal, intraocular, subretinal, and intravenous. Patients will be followed for 12 months with serial comprehensive eye examinations, including relevant imaging and diagnostic ophthalmic testing.

J. N. Weiss, *Clinical Trials in Retinitis Pigmentosa Treatment*,
https://doi.org/10.1007/978-3-031-58799-3_5

Official Title
Bone-Marrow-Derived Stem Cell Ophthalmology Treatment Study II

Conditions
Retinal Disease
Age-Related Macular Degeneration
Retinitis Pigmentosa
Stargardt Disease
14 More Conditions

Intervention/Treatment
Procedure: Arm 1

Study Start (Actual)
2016-01

Primary Completion (Estimated)
2024-07

Study Completion (Estimated)
2025-07

Enrollment (Estimated)
500

Study Type
Interventional

Phase
Not Applicable

Other Study ID Numbers
SCOTS2

Eligibility Criteria
Inclusion Criteria

- Have objective, documented damage to the retina or optic nerve unlikely to improve OR
- Have objective, documented damage to the retina or optic nerve that is progressive AND have less than or equal to 20/30 best corrected central visual acuity in one or both eyes AND/OR an abnormal visual field in one or both eyes.
- Be at least 3-month post-surgical treatment intended to treat any ophthalmologic disease and stable.
- If under current medical therapy (pharmacologic treatment) for a retinal or optic nerve disease be considered stable on that treatment and unlikely to have visual function improvement (for example, glaucoma with intraocular pressure stable on topical medications but visual field damage).
- Have the potential for improvement with BMSC treatment and be at minimal risk of any potential harm from the procedure.

- Be over the age of 18
- Be medically stable and able to be medically cleared by their primary care physician or a licensed primary care practitioner for the procedure.
- Medical clearance means that in the estimation of the primary care practitioner, the patient can reasonably be expected to undergo the procedure without significant medical risk to health.

Exclusion Criteria

- Patients who are not capable of an adequate ophthalmologic examination or evaluation to document the pathology.
- Patients who are not capable or not willing to undergo follow-up eye exams with the Principal Investigator or their ophthalmologist or optometrist as outlined in the protocol.
- Patients who are not capable of providing informed consent.
- Patients who may be at significant risk to general health or to the eyes and visual function should they undergo the procedure.

Ages Eligible for Study

18 years and older (Adult, Older Adult)

Sexes Eligible for Study

All

Accepts Healthy Volunteers

No

General Publications

- Weiss JN, Levy S. The Role of Patient Funded Clinical Research in Advancing Medical Care. ClinicalTrials.gov Identifier: NCT01920867.
- Weiss JN, Levy S, Malkin A. Stem Cell Ophthalmology Treatment Study (SCOTS) for Retinal and Optic Nerve Disease: a Preliminary Report. Neural Regeneration Research. 10;6: 982–988, 2015.
- Weiss JN, Levy S, Benes SC. Stem Cell Ophthalmology Treatment Study (SCOTS) for Retina and Optic Nerve Disease: Case Report of Improvement in Relapsing Auto-Immune Optic Neuropathy. Neural Regeneration Research. 10;9:1507–1515, 2015.
- Weiss JN, Benes SC, Levy S. Stem Cell Ophthalmology Treatment Study (SCOTS): Improvement in Serpiginous Choroidopathy following Autologous Bone Marrow Derived Stem Cells. Neural Regeneration Research 11:1512–1516, 2016.
- Weiss JN, Benes SC, Levy S. Stem Cell Ophthalmology Treatment Study (SCOTS): Bone Marrow Derived Stem Cells in the Treatment of Lebers Hereditary Optic Neuropathy. Neural Regeneration Research. 11:1685–1694, 2016.
- Weiss JN, Levy S. Neurologic Stem Cell Treatment Study (NEST) using bone marrow derived stem cells for the treatment of neurological disorders and injuries: study protocol for a nonrandomized efficacy trial. Clin Transl Degener Dis. 12;1(4):176–180, 2016.

- Weiss JN, Benes SC, Levy S. Stem Cell Ophthalmology Treatment Study: bone marrow derived stem cells in the treatment of non-arteritic ischemic optic neuropathy (NAION). Stem Cell Investigation. November 2017. http://sci.amegroups.com/issue/view/632.
- Weiss JN, Levy S. Autologous bone-marrow derived stem cells in the treatment of "untreatable" optic nerve and retinal conditions. EC Ophthalmology 9.5(2018):332–336.
- Weiss JN, Levy S. Stem Cell Ophthalmology Treatment Study: bone marrow derived stem cells in the treatment of Retinitis Pigmentosa. Stem Cell Investigation https://doi.org/10.21037/sci.2018.04.02.
- Weiss JN, Levy S. Dynamic Light Scattering Spectroscopy of the Retina – A non-invasive quantitative technique to objectively document visual improvement following ocular stem cell treatment. Stem Cell Investig. 2019;6:8 https://doi.org/10.21037/sci.2019.03.01.
- Weiss JN, Levy S. Stem Cell Ophthalmology Treatment Study (SCOTS): Bone marrow derived stem cells in the treatment of Usher syndrome. Stem Cell Investig. 2019;9:9 https://doi.org/10.21037/sci.2019.08.07.
- Weiss JN, Levy S. Stem Cell Ophthalmology Treatment Study (SCOTS): Autologous bone-marrow derived stem cells in the treatment of hereditary macular degeneration. EC Ophthalmology 10.7 (2019): 536–542.
- Weiss JN, Levy S. Stem Cell Ophthalmology Treatment Study (SCOTS): Bone marrow derived stem cells in the treatment of Dominant Optic Atrophy. Stem Cell Investig. 2019; https://doi.org/10.21037/sci.2019.11.01.
- Weiss JN, Levy S. Stem Cell Ophthalmology Treatment Study (SCOTS): Bone marrow derived stem cells in the treatment of Age-related Macular Degeneration. Medicines 2020, 7,16; https://doi.org/10.3390/medicines7040016,1-13.
- Weiss, JN, Levy, S. Stem Cell Ophthalmology Treatment Study (SCOTS): Bone Marrow-Derived Stem Cells in the Treatment of Stargardt Disease. Medicines 2021, 8, 10. https://doi.org/10.3390/medicines8020010,1-10.
- Weiss JN, Levy S. Stem Cell Ophthalmology Treatment Study: bone marrow derived stem cells in the treatment of Retinitis Pigmentosa. Stem Cell Investigation. https://doi.org/10.21037/sci.2018.04.02.
- Weiss JN, Levy S. Stem Cell Ophthalmology Treatment Study (SCOTS): Bone marrow derived stem cells in the treatment of Usher syndrome. Stem Cell Investig. 2019;6:31. http://sci.amegroups.com/article/view/29013/html

Abstract Background: Seventeen patients with bilateral visual loss due to retinitis pigmentosa (RP) underwent autologous bone-marrow-derived stem cell (BMSC) treatment within the Stem Cell Ophthalmology Treatment Study (SCOTS and SCOTS 2). Both are National Institutes of Health and Office of Human Research Protection compliant Institutional Review Board approved clinical studies utilizing using autologous BMSC in the treatment of retinal and optic nerve diseases that meet inclusion criteria.

Methods: The average age of the patients treated was 48.8 years. The average duration of disease prior to treatment was 27.6 years and ranged from 4 to approximately 60 years. Affected eyes were treated with either retrobulbar, subtenon, and intravenous BMSC or retrobulbar, subtenon, intravitreal, and intravenous. Follow-up was provided a minimum of 6 months. The primary outcome was visual acuity as measured by Snellen or converted to LogMAR.

Results: Following therapy in SCOTS or SCOTS 2, 11 patients (64.7%) showed improved binocular vision averaging 10.23 lines of Snellen acuity per eye over pre-treatment acuity; 8 patients (35.3%) remaining stable over the follow-up period; no patients experiencing loss of overall acuity. In 33 treated eyes, 15 eyes (45.5%) improved an average of 7.9 lines of Snellen acuity, 15 eyes (45.5%) remained stable, and 3 eyes (9%) worsened by an average of 1.7 lines of Snellen acuity. Improvements ranged from 1 to 27 lines of vision. Using the Logmar Scale and calculating delta as a ratio to pre-treatment vision in improved eyes, acuity improvement ranged from 23% to 90% with an average of 40.9% visual acuity improvement over baseline vision. Evaluation of all patients and eyes capable of LogMAR vision showed an average of 31% improvement in vision over baseline. Findings were of statistical significance ($p = 0.016$). There were no surgical complications.

Conclusions: The BMSC protocols of the Stem Cell Ophthalmology Treatment Study achieved meaningful visual acuity improvements or stability in RP that were of statistical significance. Duration of disease did not appear to affect the ability of eyes to respond. Safety was confirmed. Possible mechanisms by which improvement occurred may include transdifferentiation of BMSC into NeuN positive cells, BMSC paracrine secretions or neurotrophic factors and hormones, transfer of mitochondria, release of messenger RNA or other compounds via exosomes or microvesicles. Given the successful outcome in this otherwise progressive condition, consideration should be given to providing this treatment option.

Abstract Background: Usher syndrome is the most common form of syndromic retinitis pigmentosa (RP) and includes types I, II, and III with varying degrees of hearing loss. We present results of ten eyes with Usher syndrome treated with autologous bone-marrow-derived stem cells (BMSC) within the Stem Cell Ophthalmology Treatment Study (SCOTS).

Methods: Preoperative Snellen visual acuities ranged from 20/30-1 to 20/400 with the average pre-operative Snellen acuity approximately 20/85 and the average logarithm of the minimum angle of resolution (LogMAR) acuity 0.635. All eyes had significantly impaired visual fields (VF) and patients reported hearing loss as part of this syndromic RP. Treatment using the protocols of the SCOTS study using BMSC provided by retrobulbar, subtenons, intravitreal, and intravenous injections.

Results: Following treatment, 80% of the Usher eyes showed an improvement in visual acuity. Of the eyes that improved the average increase in visual acuity was 36.4% on LogMAR with improvements ranging from 23% to 94%. The average post-operative change in all treated eyes was a gain of 0.18 LogMAR and an increase in visual acuity of 28.3% on LogMAR. The results showed high statistical significance with $p < 0.001$. VF generally improved. No patient experienced a loss of vision. One patient underwent preoperative and 4-month post-operative audiometry testing which demonstrated improvement. The procedures were performed safely and without complications.

Conclusions: Findings confirm meaningful improvement in visual acuity is possible in Usher syndrome using BMSC protocols developed in the SCOTS study. Statistical significance and safety were established.

Recruiting

United States

CNS10-NPC for the Treatment of RP

ClinicalTrials.gov ID NCT04284293

Sponsor Cedars-Sinai Medical Center
Information provided by Clive Svendsen, Cedars-Sinai Medical Center (Responsible Party)
Last Update Posted 2023-02-13

Brief Summary
The investigator is examining the safety of transplanting cells into the subretinal space of patients with RP. The cells are called neural progenitor cells, which are a type of stem cell that can become several different types of cells in the nervous system. These cells have been derived to specifically become astrocytes, which is a type of neuronal cell. The cells are called "CNS10-NPC." The investigational treatment has been tested in animals, but it has not yet been tested in people. In this study, the investigators want to learn if CNS10-NPC cells are safe to transplant into the subretinal space of people.

Detailed Description
This study will be the first to use a human progenitor cell line to treat RP in people. This is a Phase 1/2a, single-center, open label, safety study of two escalating doses of human neural progenitor cells (CNS10-NPC) delivered unilaterally to the subretinal space of subjects with RP.

Subjects meeting all Eligibility Criteria and providing Informed Consent will be enrolled in one of the two sequential dosing groups. Subjects will be treated sequentially with a minimum of 1-month interval between surgeries for the first three subjects in each dosing cohort. The remaining subjects in the cohort will be treated with a minimum interval of at least 1 week between surgeries.

Primary Objective To assess the safety and tolerability of two escalating doses of clinical grade human fetal cortical-derived neural progenitor cells (CNS10-NPC) administered in the subretinal space of one eye (unilaterally) in patients with RP.

Secondary Objectives Within constraints of a small first in-human study focused on safety:

1. Determine if CNS10-NPC can engraft and survive long term in the retina of transiently immunosuppressed subjects,
2. Obtain evidence that subretinal injection of CNS10-NPC can favorably impact the progression of vision loss in subjects with moderate RP.

Official Title
Clinical Study to Assess Safety and Efficacy of Subretinal Injection of Human Neural Progenitor Cells for Treatment of Retinitis Pigmentosa

Conditions
Retinitis Pigmentosa

Study Type
Interventional

Enrollment (Estimated)
16

Intervention/Treatment
Biological: CNS10-NPC implantation

Phase
Phase 1

Other Study Id Numbers
Study 00000375

Study Start (Actual)
2021-07-22

Primary Completion (Estimated)
2024-11

Study Completion (Estimated)
2024-11
Study Contact
Name: Pablo Avalos, MD
Phone Number: 310-248-8584
Email: Pablo.Avalos@cshs.org
United States

Beverly Hills, California, United States, 90211
Recruiting
Retina-Vitreous Associates Medical Group

Contact
Janet Kurokouchi
310-289-2478 ext. 3 jkurokouchi@laretina.com
Principal Investigator:
David Liao, MD, PhD

Eligibility Criteria
Ages Eligible For Study
18 Years and older (Adult, Older Adult)

Accepts Healthy Volunteer
No

Sexes Eligible For Study
All

Description

Inclusion Criteria
- To participate in this study, the subject must be 18 years of age or older and must understand and sign the protocol's informed consent.
- Participant with diagnosis of retinitis pigmentosa.
  - Clinical signs of retinitis pigmentosa.
  - A history of nyctalopia
  - Retinal pigmentary changes
  - Arteriolar attenuation
  - Waxy disc pallor
  - Electrophysiologic evidence of rod dysfunction on full field electroretinography
  - Visual field constriction.
- (a) Participants in Group 1 ($n = 6$) will have visual acuity equal to or worse than 20/200. Participants in Group 2 ($n = 10$) will have visual acuity equal to or worse than 20/80.
- (b) Group 1 participants will have central visual field of 40° diameter or less. Group 2, participants will have a measurable visual field defect.
- Participant will be medically able to undergo ophthalmic surgery.

Exclusion Criteria
- Presence of significant ocular abnormalities that would preclude the planned surgery or interfere with the interpretation of study endpoints (e.g., glaucoma, corneal or significant lens opacities, pre-existing uveitis, intraocular infection, macular edema, and choroidal neovascularization). Any ocular diseases that the investigator feels would interfere with accurate ocular measurements. This would exclude potential subjects with significant cataract, corneal scars, or significant corneal irregularities, such as keratoconus, previous penetrating keratoplasty or glaucoma with central visual field.
- Any pre-existing factor or history of eye disease that may predispose to an increased risk of surgical complications in the study eye (e.g., trauma, previous surgery other than uncomplicated cataract surgery, uveitis, and congenital developmental or structural abnormalities).

- Concomitant systemic diseases including those in which the disease itself, or the treatment for the disease, can alter ocular function or immune status (e.g., malignancies, uncontrolled diabetes).
- Any ocular surgery or laser in either eye within 12 weeks of screening.
- Any contraindication to pupil dilatation in either eye.
- Treatment with intravitreal, subtenon or periocular steroid within 4 months of enrollment.
- Any known allergy to any component of the delivery vehicle or diagnostic agents used during the study (e.g., dilation drops), or medications planned for use during the peri-operative period, including corticosteroids, tacrolimus, and mycophenolate.
- Imminently life-threatening illness.
- Abuse of alcohol or any illegal substance(s) within 12 months of the procedure.
- Laboratory test abnormalities or abnormalities in electrocardiogram or chest X-ray, which in the opinion of the Principal Investigator, are clinically significant and would make the patient unable to tolerate study procedures.
- Intercurrent illness or infection 28 days prior to enrolment.
- Contraindications to use of anesthesia.
- Females of child-bearing potential (e.g., those who are not surgically sterile and not at least 12-month post-menopausal) who are not willing to comply with the study's contraception requirement (women who are unwilling to use an effective form of contraception such as the contraceptive pill or intrauterine device).
- Women who are pregnant.
- Females who are nursing or who intend to nurse during the first 6-month post-treatment.
- Men or women who do not agree to use barrier or medical contraception for at least 6 months post-operatively.
- History of any investigational agent administration within 28 days prior to administration.
- Participation in a prior gene transfer therapy study or cell-based therapy.
- Enrollment in any other clinical study, for any condition, including those relating to RP throughout the duration of the study.
- Current or anticipated long-term treatment with systemic corticosteroids (for a period longer than 7 days).
- Current treatment with immunosuppressant therapies or any contraindications to use of the immunosuppressants in this protocol.
- A history of malignancy within a 5-year period or a positive cancer screening test within a 1-year period of the screening visit.
- Any physical or mental disability that will impair the ability of the patient to travel to and from the study center or provide informed consent/assent or effective safety assessments as specified by the protocol. Any mental or psychiatric disorders that prevent the patient from having full authority to do so (e.g., the subject cannot have power of attorney signed over to another individual).
- Inability or unwillingness to comply with the study protocol.
- Medical history of HIV, or hepatitis A, B or C.

- Subjects who have taken any prescription or investigational oral retinoid medication (e.g., Accutane® Soriatane®), or any medicines that may affect the macula (e.g., tamoxifen, mellaril, thorazine, plaquenil, and niacin) within 6 months of enrollment.
- Allergy to Beta-Lactam antibiotics.
- The presence of cystoid macular edema.
- Glucose-6-phosphate dehydrogenase (G6PD) Deficiency

Design Details

Primary Purpose: Treatment
Allocation: Non-Randomized
Interventional Model: Sequential Assignment
Masking: None (Open Label)

Arms and interventions

Participant group/arm	Intervention/treatment
Experimental: Group 1A Visual acuity of 20/200 or worse Single, unilateral, subretinal injection of 300,000 CNS10-NPC ($n = 3$)	Biological: CNS10-NPC implantation • All patients will receive a single, unilateral, subretinal injection of CNS10-NPC • Other Names: – Neural Progenitor Cell (NPC) – Stem Cell
Experimental: Group 1B Visual acuity of 20/200 or worse Single, unilateral, subretinal injection of 1,000,000 CNS10-NPC ($n = 3$)	Biological: CNS10-NPC implantation • All patients will receive a single, unilateral, subretinal injection of CNS10-NPC • Other Names: – Neural Progenitor Cell (NPC) – Stem Cell
Experimental: Group 2 Visual acuity between 20/80 and 20/200 Single, unilateral, subretinal injection of 1,000,000 CNS10-NPC ($n = 10$)	Biological: CNS10-NPC implantation • All patients will receive a single, unilateral, subretinal injection of CNS10-NPC • Other Names: – Neural Progenitor Cell (NPC) – Stem Cell

Primary outcome measures

Outcome measure	Measure description	Time frame
Safety as evaluated by incidence of Adverse Events (AE) and Serious Adverse Events (SAE) and their relationship to the intervention		Subjects will be followed postoperatively for 12 months
Safety, as evaluated by changes in the complete blood count		Subjects will be followed postoperatively for 12 months
Safety, as evaluated by changes in the comprehensive metabolic panel		Subjects will be followed postoperatively for 12 months

Safety, as evaluated by changes in Donor Specific Antibodies		Subjects will be followed postoperatively for 12 months
Safety, as evaluated by changes in the urinalysis		Subjects will be followed postoperatively for 12 months
Safety, as evaluated by changes in Visual Acuity	ETDRS, or FrACT in cases of very low vision	Subjects will be followed postoperatively for 12 months
Safety, as evaluated by changes in visual field	Goldman perimetry will be used for central visual fields and microperimetry will be used for peripheral visual fields	Subjects will be followed postoperatively for 12 months
Safety, as evaluated by changes in Spectral Domain Optical Coherence Tomography (SD-OCT)	Ellipsoid zone measurement through SD-OCT will be performed	Subjects will be followed postoperatively for 12 months

Secondary outcome measures

Outcome measure	Measure description	Time frame
Slit lamp examination		Performed 7 times over 15 months
Intraocular pressure measurement		Performed 7 times over 15 months
Funduscopic examination		Performed 7 times over 15 months
Fundus photography (color, red free, or infrared)		Performed 4 times over 15 months
Fundus Autofluorescence (FAF)		Performed 4 times over 15 months
Best Corrected Visual Acuity		Performed 7 times over 15 months
Visual Function Questionnaire-25 (VFQ-25)	The Visual Function Questionnaire-25 is graded in a scale from 0 to 100 where a higher number represents better function	Performed 5 times over 15 months
Spectral domain optical coherence tomography (SD-OCT)	Retinal Thickness	Performed 5 times over 15 months
Electroretinography (ERG)		Performed 5 times over 15 months
Goldmann visual field area (microperimetry)		Performed 5 times over 15 months
Change in rate of vision field loss		Through study completion, ~15 months.

Sponsor
Cedars-Sinai Medical Center

Collaborators
- California Institute for Regenerative Medicine (CIRM)

Investigators
- Principal Investigator: David Liao, MD, PhD, Retina-Vitreous Associates Medical Group

General Publications
No publications available

Discussion
The concern is whether the cells are able to engraft and function. Engrafting without function is of no benefit. As the Jcyte studies have shown, the loss of too many rods prevents the cones from functioning.

Recruiting

Caribbean/Argentina/Mexico

Safety of Cultured Allogeneic Adult Umbilical Cord-Derived Mesenchymal Stem Cells for Eye Diseases

ClinicalTrials.gov ID NCT05147701

Sponsor The Foundation for Orthopedics and Regenerative Medicine
Information provided by The Foundation for Orthopedics and Regenerative Medicine (Responsible Party)
Last Update Posted 2022-10-27

Brief Summary
This trial will study the safety and efficacy of intravenous and sub-tenon delivery of cultured allogeneic adult umbilical cord-derived mesenchymal stem cells for the treatment of eye diseases.

Detailed Description
This patient funded trial aims to study the safety and efficacy of intravenous and sub-tenon delivery of cultured allogeneic adult umbilical cord-derived mesenchymal stem cells (UC-MSCs) for the treatment of eye diseases. The total dose will be 100 million cells. Patients will be evaluated within 1-month pre-treatment, and at 1-, 6-, 12-, 24-, 36-, and 48-month post-treatment for safety and efficacy.

For patients with more severe disease, an autologous effector cells (activated lymphocytes) treatment will be utilized created from the patient's own cells obtained by apheresis.

Official Title
Safety of Cultured Allogeneic Adult Umbilical Cord-Derived Mesenchymal Stem Cells for the Treatment of Eye Diseases

Conditions
Eye Diseases
Retinitis Pigmentosa
Glaucoma
Diabetic Retinopathy
Macular Degeneration
Traumatic Optic Neuropathy
Optic Atrophy

Study Type
Interventional

Enrollment (Estimated)
20

Intervention/Treatment
Biological: AlloRx

Phase
Phase 1

Other Study ID Numbers
ATG-1-MSC-014

Study Start (Actual)
2022-02-01

Primary Completion (Estimated)
2026-01

Study Completion (Estimated)
Antigua and Barbuda

St. John's, Antigua and Barbuda
Recruiting
Medical Surgical Associates Center

Contact
Chadwick Prodromos, M.D.
8476996810 care@thepsci.com

Argentina

Buenos Aires, Argentina
Recruiting
Center for Investigation in Tissue Engineering and Cellular Therapy

Contact
Chadwick Prodromos, M.D.
8476996810 ext. 202 Care@thepsci.com

Mexico
N.L Locations

San Pedro Garza García, N.L, Mexico
Recruiting
Medyca Bosques

Contact
Chadwick Prodromos, M.D.
8476996810 ext. 202 Care@thepsci.com

Eligibility Criteria
Ages Eligible For Study
(Child, Adult, Older Adult)

Accepts Healthy Volunteer
No

Sexes Eligible For Study
All

Description

Inclusion Criteria
- Diagnosis of eye disease
- Understanding and willingness to sign a written informed consent document

Exclusion Criteria
- Active infection
- Active cancer
- Chronic multisystem organ failure
- Pregnancy
- Clinically significant Abnormalities on pre-treatment laboratory evaluation
- Medical condition that would (based on the opinion of the investigator) compromise patient's safety
- Continued drug abuse
- Pre-menopausal women not using contraception
- Previous organ transplant
- Hypersensitivity to sulfur

Primary Purpose: Treatment
Allocation: N/A
Interventional Model: Single Group Assignment
Masking: None (Open Label)

Arms and interventions

Participant group/arm	Intervention/treatment
Experimental: Treatment Group (AlloRx) intravenous and sub-tenon delivery (total dose of 100 million cells)	Biological: AlloRx • cultured allogeneic adult umbilical cord-derived mesenchymal stem cells

Primary outcome measures

Outcome measure	Measure description	Time frame
Safety (adverse events)	Clinical monitoring of possible adverse events or complications	Four-year follow-up

Sponsor

The Foundation for Orthopedics and Regenerative Medicine

Collaborators

No information provided

Investigators

- Principal Investigator: Chadwick Prodromos, MD, The Foundation for Orthopedics and Regenerative Medicine

General Publications

- Sung Y, Lee SM, Park M, Choi HJ, Kang S, Choi BI, Lew H. Treatment of traumatic optic neuropathy using human placenta-derived mesenchymal stem cells in Asian patients. Regen Med. 2020 Oct;15(10):2163–2179. https://doi.org/10.2217/rme-2020-0044. Epub 2020 Dec 14.
- Zhao T, Liang Q, Meng X, Duan P, Wang F, Li S, Liu Y, Yin ZQ. Intravenous Infusion of Umbilical Cord Mesenchymal Stem Cells Maintains and Partially Improves Visual Function in Patients with Advanced Retinitis Pigmentosa. Stem Cells Dev. 2020 Aug;29(16):1029–1037. https://doi.org/10.1089/scd.2020.0037. Epub 2020 Jul 15.
- Ozmert E, Arslan U. Management of retinitis pigmentosa by Wharton's jelly derived mesenchymal stem cells: preliminary clinical results. Stem Cell Res Ther. 2020 Jan 13;11(1):25. https://doi.org/10.1186/s13287-020-1549-6.

Discussion

The Principal Investigator is an orthopedic surgeon. No mention is made of who will be performing the subtenon injection. However, the basic question to be answered is important. Will the results with umbilical cord-derived cells be non-inferior to those results obtained with the present gold standard, autologous BMSC?

Recruiting

Turkey

The Effect of Stem Cells and Stem Cell Exosomes on Visual Functions in Patients with Retinitis Pigmentosa

ClinicalTrials.gov ID NCT05413148

Sponsor TC Erciyes University
Information provided by Kuddusi Erkılıç, TC Erciyes University (Responsible Party)
Last Update Posted 2022-09-07

Brief Summary
This clinical trial aims to study the efficacy of umbilical cord-derived mesenchymal stem cells and their exosomes in the treatment of RP . The participants will be randomized into three groups. Functional and structural parameters will be compared before and after the injections and also will be compared among the groups to reveal whether stem cell and their exosomes are more effective than placebo.

Detailed Description
RP is one of the leading causes of vision loss and irreversible blindness. It is stated that 1.4 million people are affected in the world and its prevalence is 1:4000. Stem cell applications are methods that are increasingly gaining importance in the field of regenerative medicine and ophthalmology. In addition to many experimental studies in retinal diseases including RP, there are also clinical studies reporting successful results on humans. The most widely used stem cell group in current clinical practice is mesenchymal stem cells. The advantages are that they are relatively easy to obtain and do not induce severe immune responses. Clinical studies in stem cell therapies for the eye suggest that stem cells benefit the surrounding tissue by secreting support such as growth factors, and extracellular vesicles, mostly due to their trophic and paracrine effects. In intraocular applications, there has been a tendency to apply mesenchymal stem cells around/outside the eye, including subtenon and suprachoroidal application due to side effects such as retinal detachment and epiretinal membrane.

Other cellular products that have been studied in animal studies and clinical research in recent years are exosomes. Exosomes are a subgroup of extracellular vesicles released from cells. Exosomes are extracellular vesicles 30–150 nm in size and carry at least one of the exosomal proteins CD63, CD9, CD81, syntenin-1 and TSG101. Exosomes are secreted from different cells in the organism and are also found in body fluids. Exosomes play a role in the transportation of biomolecules, such as lipids, carbohydrates, nucleic acids, and proteins from one cell to another, and in this way, they function in genetic information transfer, and reprogramming of the opposite cell and intercellular communication. One of the sources of exosomes is mesenchymal stem cells that secrete high amounts of exosomes. Mesenchymal stem cell-derived exosomes have been reported to have therapeutic effects, just like mesenchymal stem cells. It is thought that stem cells also exert their clinical effects through paracrine factors they secrete rather than being implanted in the tissue. However, the mechanism of action of mesenchymal stem cells has not been fully understood, and exosomes are thought to contribute to the effect. The storage and durability of exosomes may provide advantages in therapeutic applications compared to mesenchymal stem cells and may provide more immunological advantages in allogeneic applications compared to cellular treatments, since they do not contain cells.

One of the sources from which mesenchymal stem cells can be obtained is Wharton jelly, which is the mesenchymal tissue of the umbilical cord. Stem cells originating from Wharton gel are a good source of stem cells due to their high differentiation capacity, high regeneration capacity, constant doubling time, high proliferation capacity, low immunogenicity, and no ethical problems due to non-invasive methods, and easy availability.

This clinical trial will enroll patients diagnosed with RP. The diagnosis of RP is made by clinical fundus examination, examinations in our clinic, and genetic analysis.

At the beginning of the study, all volunteers will undergo a full ophthalmologic examination, including best-corrected visual acuity, anterior segment and fundus examination with a slit lamp, optical coherence tomography (OCT), visual field (VF), electroretinogram (ERG), multifocal ERG (mfERG), and optical coherence tomography (OCTA). Retinal and choroidal thickness and ellipsoid bandwidth in OCT, MD (mean deviation) value showing sensitivity in VF, amplitude and latency times in ERG and mf-ERG, vascular density, and vascular flow ratios in OCTA will be recorded.

The volunteers will be randomized into three groups. The first group will be the placebo group (45 volunteers) and 0.5 cc saline physiological saline will be applied to the subtenon space. Second group of patients (45 volunteers) will undergo a subtenon injection of Wharton gel-derived mesenchymal stem cell suspension. A suspension containing mesenchymal stem cell exosomes from Wharton jelly will be applied to the subtenon distance to the third group of patients (45 volunteers). A single eye of each volunteer will be included. Informed consent will be obtained from the volunteers.

Allogeneic human Wharton gel tissue-derived mesenchymal stem cells and their exosomes will be obtained from healthy female volunteers, who is over 18 years, under sterile conditions after HBV, HCV, HIV virus, and "Treponema Pallidum" (VDRL) tests were performed. Cord tissue obtained from birth will be carried in a sterile transfer solution and will be processed to obtain stem cells in Erciyes University Genome and Stem Cell GMP (good manufacturing practices) certified laboratories. Exosomes will be obtained by the ultracentrifugation method in the same facility.

For injection into the subtenon space, the conjunctiva and tenon will be opened with a small incision about 10 mm away from the lower temporal area, then 20 gauge curved subtenon cannula will be advanced parallel to the sclera and injected into the posterior subtenon area. All volunteers will be prescribed antibiotics and steroid drops after the surgical procedure.

Full ophthalmological examination and examinations at the beginning of the study will be performed and recorded again on the first day, first month, second month, third month, and sixth month of the anterior segment and fundus examination, OCT, VF, ERG, mfERG, and OCTA examinations will be performed.

In addition, a questionnaire evaluating the visual functions subjectively will be administered at the first-, third-, and sixth-month visits. (National Eye Institute Visual Functioning Questionnaire–25/National Eye Institute (USA) Visual Function Questionnaire). Two masked investigators will perform analyses.

Post-procedure first-day, first-month, second-month, third-month and sixth-month data will be compared among study groups and within groups.

Official Title
The Effect of Wharton Jelly-Derived Mesenchymal Stem Cells and Stem Cell Exosomes on Visual Functions in Patients with Retinitis Pigmentosa

Conditions
Retinitis Pigmentosa

Study Type
Interventional

Enrollment (Estimated)
135

Intervention/Treatment
Biological: Subtenon injection of Wharton jelly-derived mesenchymal stem cells
Biological: Subtenon injection of Wharton jelly-derived mesenchymal stem cell exosomes
Other: Placebo

Phase
Phase 2 Phase 3

Other Study ID Numbers
TSG-2021-11599

Study Start (Actual)
2022-08-05

Primary Completion (Estimated)
2023-07-01

Study Completion (Estimated)
2023-12-15

Study Contact
Name: Osman Ahmet POLAT, MD
Phone Number: 905424395196
Email: osmanahmet@gmail.com
Turkey

Kayseri, Turkey, 38039
Recruiting
Erciyes University, Faculty of Medicine

Contact
OSMAN AHMET POLAT, MD
+905424395196 osmanpolat@erciyes.edu.tr

Eligibility Criteria
Ages Eligible For Study
18–70 Years (Adult, Older Adult)
Accepts Healthy Volunteer
No
Sexes Eligible For Study
All

Description

Inclusion Criteria
- 18 years and over
- Diagnosis of RP: by clinical history, fundus examination, visual field (GA), electroretinogram (ERG), and genetic analysis
- Visual field loss
- The best corrected visual acuity of 0.05 on the Snellen chart
- The MD (mean deviation) value in the visual field is between 33.0 and −5.0 dB
- Intraocular pressure value below 22 mmHg

Exclusion Criteria
- Presence of cataracts or other media opacities that may affect imaging and tests
- Diagnosis of glaucoma
- History of ocular surgery or injection in the last 6 months
- Visual level too low for examinations (0.05 and below)
- Diagnosis of any systemic disease (such as diabetes, uncontrolled hypertension, and neurological disease)
- Smoking and substance abuse

Design Details
Primary Purpose: Treatment
Allocation: Randomized
Interventional Model: Parallel Assignment
Masking: Triple (Participant Investigator Outcomes Assessor)

Arms and interventions

Participant group/arm	Intervention/treatment
Active Comparator: Wharton jelly-derived mesenchymal stem cell Single subtenon injection of Wharton jelly-derived mesenchymal stem cells will be performed on a single eye after randomization	Biological: Subtenon injection of Wharton jelly-derived mesenchymal stem cells • Single subtenon injection for single eye
Active Comparator: Mesenchymal stem cell exosome (Wharton jelly-derived) Single subtenon injection of mesenchymal stem cell exosomes (Wharton jelly-derived) will be performed on a single eye after randomization.	Biological: Subtenon injection of Wharton jelly-derived mesenchymal stem cell exosomes • Single subtenon injection for single eye
Placebo Comparator: Placebo A single subtenon injection of saline will be performed on a single eye after randomization.	Other: Placebo • Single Subtenon injection of saline for a single eye

Primary outcome measures

Outcome measure	Measure description	Time frame
Evaluation of best corrected visual acuity change	Visual acuity change with LogMar Chart	Up to 6 months
Evaluation of visual field change	Mean deviation values of automatic visual field testing	Up to 6 months

Secondary outcome measures

Outcome measure	Measure description	Time frame
Evaluation of multifocal ERG changes	Amplitudes changes in multifocal ERG testing	Up to 6 months
Evaluation of ERG changes	Amplitude changes in multifocal ERG testing	Up to 6 months
Evaluation of optical coherence tomography changes	Retinal thickness changes in optical coherence tomography change	Up to 6 months
Evaluation of optical coherence tomography angiography changes	Vascular density changes in optical coherence tomography angiography	Up to 6 months

Sponsor

TC Erciyes University

Collaborators

No information provided

Investigators

- Principal Investigator: Kuddusi ERKILIÇ, Professor, Erciyes University Medical Faculty

General Publications

- Limoli PG, Limoli CSS, Morales MU, Vingolo EM. Mesenchymal stem cell surgery, rescue and regeneration in retinitis pigmentosa: clinical and rehabilitative prognostic aspects. Restor Neurol Neurosci. 2020;38(3):223–237. https://doi.org/10.3233/RNN-190970.

- Bhattacharya S, Gangaraju R, Chaum E. Recent Advances in Retinal Stem Cell Therapy. Curr Mol Biol Rep. 2017 Sep;3(3):172–182. https://doi.org/10.1007/s40610-017-0069-3. Epub 2017 Jul 10.
- Limoli PG, Vingolo EM, Limoli C, Nebbioso M. Stem Cell Surgery and Growth Factors in Retinitis Pigmentosa Patients: Pilot Study after Literature Review. Biomedicines. 2019 Nov 30;7(4):94. https://doi.org/10.3390/biomedicines7040094.
- Borkowska-Kuczkowska A, Slugocka D, Swiatkowska-Flis B, Boruczkowski D. The use of mesenchymal stem cells for the treatment of progressive retinal diseases: a review. Regen Med. 2019 May;14(4):321–329. https://doi.org/10.2217/rme-2019-0022. Epub 2019 Apr 12.
- Jin ZB, Gao ML, Deng WL, Wu KC, Sugita S, Mandai M, Takahashi M. Stemming retinal regeneration with pluripotent stem cells. Prog Retin Eye Res. 2019 Mar;69:38–56. https://doi.org/10.1016/j.preteyeres.2018.11.003. Epub 2018 Nov 9.
- Ozmert E, Arslan U. Management of retinitis pigmentosa by Wharton's jelly derived mesenchymal stem cells: preliminary clinical results. Stem Cell Res Ther. 2020 Jan 13;11(1):25. https://doi.org/10.1186/s13287-020-1549-6.
- Oner A. Stem Cell Treatment in Retinal Diseases: Recent Developments. Turk J Ophthalmol. 2018 Feb;48(1):33–38. doi: https://doi.org/10.4274/tjo.89972. Epub 2018 Feb 23.
- Cotrim CC, Jorge R, Oliveira MC, Pieroni F, Messias AMV, Siqueira RC. Clinical studies using stem cells for treatment of retinal diseases: state of the art. Arq Bras Oftalmol. 2020 Mar-Apr;83(2):160–167. https://doi.org/10.5935/0004-2749.20200037.
- Huo DM, Dong FT, Yu WH, Gao F. Differentiation of mesenchymal stem cell in the microenvironment of retinitis pigmentosa. Int J Ophthalmol. 2010;3(3):216–9. https://doi.org/10.3980/j.issn.2222-3959.2010.03.08. Epub 2010 Sep 18.
- Satarian L, Nourinia R, Safi S, Kanavi MR, Jarughi N, Daftarian N, Arab L, Aghdami N, Ahmadieh H, Baharvand H. Intravitreal Injection of Bone Marrow Mesenchymal Stem Cells in Patients with Advanced Retinitis Pigmentosa; a Safety Study. J Ophthalmic Vis Res. 2017 Jan-Mar;12(1):58–64. https://doi.org/10.4103/2008-322X.200164.
- Kuriyan AE, Albini TA, Townsend JH, Rodriguez M, Pandya HK, Leonard RE second, Parrott MB, Rosenfeld PJ, Flynn HW Jr., Goldberg JL. Vision Loss after Intravitreal Injection of Autologous "Stem Cells" for AMD. N Engl J Med. 2017 Mar 16;376(11):1047–1053. https://doi.org/10.1056/NEJMoa1609583.
- Harrell CR, Fellabaum C, Jovicic N, Djonov V, Arsenijevic N, Volarevic V. Molecular Mechanisms Responsible for Therapeutic Potential of Mesenchymal Stem Cell-Derived Secretome. Cells. 2019 May 16;8(5):467. https://doi.org/10.3390/cells8050467.
- Klingeborn M, Dismuke WM, Bowes Rickman C, Stamer WD. Roles of exosomes in the normal and diseased eye. Prog Retin Eye Res. 2017 Jul;59:158–177. https://doi.org/10.1016/j.preteyeres.2017.04.004. Epub 2017 Apr 29.

- Harrell CR, Simovic Markovic B, Fellabaum C, Arsenijevic A, Djonov V, Arsenijevic N, Volarevic V. Therapeutic Potential of Mesenchymal Stem Cell-Derived Exosomes in the Treatment of Eye Diseases. Adv Exp Med Biol. 2018;1089:47–57. https://doi.org/10.1007/5584_2018_219.
- Mead B, Tomarev S. Extracellular vesicle therapy for retinal diseases. Prog Retin Eye Res. 2020 Nov;79:100849. https://doi.org/10.1016/j.preteyeres.2020.100849. Epub 2020 Mar 10.
- Yaghoubi Y, Movassaghpour A, Zamani M, Talebi M, Mehdizadeh A, Yousefi M. Human umbilical cord mesenchymal stem cells derived-exosomes in diseases treatment. Life Sci. 2019 Sep 15;233:116733. https://doi.org/10.1016/j.lfs.2019.116733. Epub 2019 Aug 5.
- Zhang X, Liu J, Yu B, Ma F, Ren X, Li X. Effects of mesenchymal stem cells and their exosomes on the healing of large and refractory macular holes. Graefes Arch Clin Exp Ophthalmol. 2018 Nov;256(11):2041–2052. https://doi.org/10.1007/s00417-018-4097-3. Epub 2018 Aug 30.
- Ma M, Li B, Zhang M, Zhou L, Yang F, Ma F, Shao H, Li Q, Li X, Zhang X. Therapeutic effects of mesenchymal stem cell-derived exosomes on retinal detachment. Exp Eye Res. 2020 Feb;191:107899. https://doi.org/10.1016/j.exer.2019.107899. Epub 2019 Dec 19.
- Yu B, Shao H, Su C, Jiang Y, Chen X, Bai L, Zhang Y, Li Q, Zhang X, Li X. Exosomes derived from MSCs ameliorate retinal laser injury partially by inhibition of MCP-1. Sci Rep. 2016 Sep 30;6:34562. https://doi.org/10.1038/srep34562.
- Zhang W, Wang Y, Kong Y. Exosomes Derived From Mesenchymal Stem Cells Modulate miR-126 to Ameliorate Hyperglycemia-Induced Retinal Inflammation Via Targeting HMGB1. Invest Ophthalmol Vis Sci. 2019 Jan 2;60(1):294–303. https://doi.org/10.1167/iovs.18-25617.
- Hajrasouliha AR, Jiang G, Lu Q, Lu H, Kaplan HJ, Zhang HG, Shao H. Exosomes from retinal astrocytes contain antiangiogenic components that inhibit laser-induced choroidal neovascularization. J Biol Chem. 2013 Sep 27;288(39):28058–67. https://doi.org/10.1074/jbc.M113.470765. Epub 2013 Aug 7.
- Ha DH, Kim SD, Lee J, Kwon HH, Park GH, Yang SH, Jung JY, Lee JH, Park SR, Youn J, Lee SH, Kim JE, Lim J, Lee HK, Cho BS, Yi YW. Toxicological evaluation of exosomes derived from human adipose tissue-derived mesenchymal stem/stromal cells. Regul Toxicol Pharmacol. 2020 Aug;115:104686. https://doi.org/10.1016/j.yrtph.2020.104686. Epub 2020 May 22.
- Pan D, Chang X, Xu M, Zhang M, Zhang S, Wang Y, Luo X, Xu J, Yang X, Sun X. UMSC-derived exosomes promote retinal ganglion cells survival in a rat model of optic nerve crush. J Chem Neuroanat. 2019 Mar;96:134–139. https://doi.org/10.1016/j.jchemneu.2019.01.006. Epub 2019 Jan 10.
- Zhao T, Liang Q, Meng X, Duan P, Wang F, Li S, Liu Y, Yin ZQ. Intravenous Infusion of Umbilical Cord Mesenchymal Stem Cells Maintains and Partially Improves Visual Function in Patients with Advanced Retinitis Pigmentosa. Stem Cells Dev. 2020 Aug;29(16):1029–1037. https://doi.org/10.1089/scd.2020.0037. Epub 2020 Jul 15.

Discussion

This study utilizes two treatment arms. The first is a subtenon injection of Wharton gel-derived mesenchymal stem cells, the second is a subtenon suspension containing mesenchymal stem cell exosomes. This study takes things a step further. Are exosomes, those non-immunogenic packages, enough to improve visual acuity? If so, then the procedure will become even easier to perform without any risk of an immunologic response.

Chapter 6
Not Yet Recruiting Stem Cell Studies

Indonesia

Role of UC-MSC and CM to Inhibit Vision Loss in Retinitis Pigmentosa Phase II/III

ClinicalTrials.gov ID NCT05909488

Sponsor PT. Prodia Stem Cell Indonesia
Information provided by PT. Prodia Stem Cell Indonesia (Responsible Party)
Last Update Posted 2023-06-18

Brief Summary
The study will perform umbilical cord-derived mesenchymal stem cell (UC-MSCs) and conditioned medium (CM) transplantation. There are two groups with different dosages. The first group will be transplanted with 1.5 million cells; meanwhile, the second group is five million cells. Each group consists of 15 subjects. All groups will be transplanted via the peribulbar route. All groups will be observed until 6 months.

Detailed Description
The eyes we will give the transplant should be given an aseptic and antiseptic technique to prevent contamination from the inside and outside. Sterile cover attached to other parts of the face except for the eyes. 1.8 ml UC-MSC preparations are suspended in CM until it reaches a 2 ml volume of cell suspension. Two dosages will be prepared, 1.5 million and five million of UC-MSC. Stem cell suspension will be injected by peribulbar, and patients will be given a quinolone antibiotic if the injection is done. On day first and day seventh after therapy, patients will be observed the presence of infection, inflammation, nd increased eye pressure. On day seventh, day 30th, and day 90th after therapy, patients will do a visual field test, visual acuity test,

J. N. Weiss, *Clinical Trials in Retinitis Pigmentosa Treatment*,
https://doi.org/10.1007/978-3-031-58799-3_6

electroretinography, funduscopy, and optical coherence tomography examination. The observations will be written in the table and analyzed by a statistic.

Study Contact
Name: dr. Muhammad B Sasongko, Sp.M, M.Epid, PhD
Phone Number: +62811293476
Email: mb.sasongko@ugm.ac.id

Study Contact Backup
Name: Dr. Cynthia R Sartika, M.Si
Email: cynthia.sartika@prostem.co.id

Eligibility Criteria

Ages Eligible For Study
18 to 65 years (Adult, Older Adult)

Accepts Healthy Volunteer
No

Sexes Eligible For Study
All

Description

Inclusion Criteria
- Vision more than 20/100
- Have more than 0.68 uV on conical receptor cell amplitude checked by ERG
- Visual field equivalent diameter more than 10o
- Willing to sign informed consent as research subjects
- Willing to do the peribulbar injection with mesenchymal stem cells isolated from umbilical cord tissue
- Willing to do visual field checks with Humphrey's perimetry, vision tests with Snellen boards, optical coherent tomography examinations, electroretinogram examinations, and fill out a quality-of-life questionnaire

Exclusion Criteria
- Pregnant or nursing women
- Positive result of HIV test
- Have a history of eye tumors
- Under immunosuppressive treatment or other drugs that can affect the growth of transplanted stem cells
- Have another eye disease such as diabetic retinopathy, uveitis, cataract, and glaucoma
- Do not come to control according to the schedule determined by the researcher (loss to follow up)

Sponsor
PT. Prodia Stem Cell Indonesia

Collaborators
No information provided

Investigators

- Principal Investigator: Dr. Muhammad B Sasongko, Sp.M, M.Epid, PhD, Gadjah Mada University, Faculty of Medicine
- Study Chair: Dr. Cosmos O Mangunsong, Sp.M, Jakarta Eye Center
- Study Chair: Dr. Rifa Widyaningrum, M.Sc, PhD, Sardjito Hospital
- Study Chair: Rima Haifa, S.Si, Prodia StemCell Indonesia
- Study Chair: Marsya N Kirana, S.T., M.Sc, Prodia StemCell Indonesia

General Publications
No publications available

Discussion
Will umbilical cord-derived stem cells produce the same or superior visual results as autologous bone-marrow-derived stem cells? This study utilizes dosages of 1.5 and 5 million cells. SCOTS utilizes more than 200 million cells. Would a similar number of umbilical cord-derived cells produce better visual results?

Chapter 7
Active, Not Recruiting Stem Cell Studies

United States

Phase 1 Study of Intravitreal Autologous CD34+ Stem Cell Therapy for Retinitis Pigmentosa (BMSCRP1)

ClinicalTrials.gov ID NCT04925687

Sponsor University of California, Davis
Information provided by Susanna Park, MD, PhD, University of California, Davis (Responsible Party)
Last Update Posted 2023-04-21

Brief Summary
In this Phase 1 open-labeled prospective study, one eye of each participant with vision loss from retinitis pigmentosa will be administered intravitreal injection of autologous CD34+ stem cells harvested from bone marrow. Each participant will be examined serially for 6 months after study injection to determine safety and feasibility of this intervention.

Official Title
Phase 1 Study of the Feasibility and Safety of Intravitreal Autologous Bone-Marrow CD34+ Stem Cell Therapy for Eyes with Vision Loss from Retinitis Pigmentosa

Conditions
Retinitis Pigmentosa

Study Type
Interventional

Enrollment (Estimated)
4

J. N. Weiss, *Clinical Trials in Retinitis Pigmentosa Treatment*,
https://doi.org/10.1007/978-3-031-58799-3_7

Intervention/Treatment
Biological: Intravitreal autologous CD34+ cells

Phase
Phase 1

Other Study ID Numbers
1743714-2

Study Start (Actual)
2021-06-01

Primary Completion (Estimated)
2023-11-30

Study Completion (Estimated)
2023-11-30

United States

Sacramento, California, United States, 95817
University of California Davis

Eligibility Criteria
Ages Eligible For Study
18 Years and older (Adult, Older Adult)

Accepts Healthy Volunteer
No

Sexes Eligible For Study
All

Inclusion Criteria
- Age > 18 years of age
- Visual Acuity at Presentation of 20/100 to Counting Fingers or constriction of peripheral visual field 360° to <10° by perimetry if BCVA is better than 20/100, duration of vision loss >3 months
- Vision loss due to retinitis pigmentosa
- The study eye has the worse visual acuity or peripheral constriction.
- Able and willing to sign consent
- Able to keep follow-up appointments for at least 6 months

Exclusion Criteria
- Other concurrent optic nerve or retinal disease in study eye affecting vision
- History of active retinal or choroidal neovascularization or macular edema in study eye requiring on-going intravitreal or periocular therapy in study eye
- Active eye or systemic infection
- Significant media opacity in the study eye precluding view of the fundus for examination, photography, or optical coherence tomography (OCT)

- Other cause for vision loss in the study eye
- History of coagulopathy or other hematologic abnormality
- Use of coumadin within 3 days of enrollment
- Concurrent immunosuppressive therapy
- History of allergy to fluorescein dye

Primary Purpose: Treatment
Allocation: N/A
Interventional Model: Single Group Assignment
Masking: None (Open Label)

Arms and interventions

Participant group/arm	Intervention/treatment
Experimental: Intravitreal autologous CD34+ cells Intravitreal injection of autologous CD34+ cells harvested from bone marrow under GMP conditions	Biological: Intravitreal autologous CD34+ cells • Autologous CD34+ cells harvested from bone-marrow-injected intravitreal

Primary outcome measures

Outcome measure	Measure description	Time frame
Safety of intravitreal injection of autologous CD34+ cells	Number and severity of Ocular and systemic adverse events	6 months
Feasibility of intravitreal injection of autologous CD34+ cells	Number of CD34+ cells harvested for intravitreal injection	Baseline

Secondary outcome measures

Outcome measure	Measure description	Time frame
Best corrected visual acuity	Change in number of letters read in study eye from baseline	6 months
Best corrected visual acuity	Change in number of letters read in study eye from baseline	1 month
Visual Field	Change in visual field area in study eye from baseline	6 months
Visual Field	Change in visual field area in study eye from baseline	1 month
Electroretinography	Change in a and b wave amplitude in study eye from baseline	6 months
Electroretinography	Change in a and b wave amplitude in study eye from baseline	1 month
National Eye Institute Vision Questionnaire	Change in Vision Questionnaire compared to baseline	6 months
National Eye Institute Vision Questionnaire	Change in Vision Questionnaire compared to baseline	1 month
Microperimetry	Change in average threshold from baseline	6 months
Microperimetry	Change percent reduced sensitivity from baseline	6 months
Microperimetry	Change in average threshold from baseline	1 month
Microperimetry	Change in percent reduced sensitivity from baseline	1 month

Sponsor
University of California, Davis

Collaborators
- Cures Within Reach
- Retina Society

Investigators
- Principal Investigator: Susanna Park, MD PhD, University of California, Davis

General Publications
No publications available

Discussion
This is the phase 1 study of the intravitreal injection of autologous bone-marrow-derived stem cells.

Active, Not Recruiting

United States

Safety and Tolerability of hRPC in Retinitis Pigmentosa (hRPCRP)

ClinicalTrials.gov ID NCT02464436

Sponsor ReNeuron Limited
Information provided by ReNeuron Limited (Responsible Party)
Last Update Posted 2023-07-06

Brief Summary
hRPC is a cell therapy for retinitis pigmentosa. This is a first-in-human, dose escalation study in which participants with retinitis pigmentosa will receive a single subretinal injection of hRPC cells in one eye to evaluate safety and tolerability.

Participants will be followed for 2 years to evaluate the safety and tolerability of hRPC Additional testing will seek to establish any preliminary efficacy from hRPC.

Detailed Description
This is a first-in-human open-label phase I/II dose-escalation study in which participants with retinitis pigmentosa will receive a single uniocular subretinal implantation of one of the three doses of hRPC.

Treated eyes will be carefully monitored for any ocular or systemic adverse events for 2 years.

Testing will comprise a series of detailed ophthalmic examinations and imaging together with blood testing and systemic evaluations, as necessary.

Ophthalmic testing will also be evaluated for any preliminary efficacy signal.

Official Title
First-In-Human Phase I/IIa, Open-Label, Prospective Study of the Safety and Tolerability of Subretinally Transplanted Human Retinal Progenitor Cells (hRPC) in Patients with Retinitis Pigmentosa (RP)

Conditions
Retinitis Pigmentosa

Study Type
Interventional

Enrollment (Actual)
29

Intervention/Treatment
Drug: hRPC

Phase
Phase 1 Phase 2

Other Study ID Numbers
RN03-CP-0001

Study Start
2015-12

Primary Completion (Actual)
2022-06

Study Completion (Estimated)
2023-12

United States

Phoenix, Arizona, United States, 85,053
Retinal Research Institute

Massachusetts Locations

Boston, Massachusetts, United States, 02114
Massachusetts Eye and Ear Infirmary

Oregon Locations

Portland, Oregon, United States, 97,239
Oregon Health and Science University

Discussion
This is the phase I/II study. I have previously commented on this work above.

Active, Not Recruiting

France

Interventional Study of Implantation of hESC-Derived RPE in Patients with RP due to Monogenic Mutation

ClinicalTrials.gov ID NCT03963154

Sponsor Centre d'Etude des Cellules Souches
Information provided by Centre d'Etude des Cellules Souches (Responsible Party)
Last Update Posted 2023-01-12

Brief Summary
Phase I/II open-label, safety, tolerability and preliminary efficacy study of implantation into one eye of human embryonic stem cell (hESC)-derived retinal pigment epithelium (RPE) in patients with retinitis pigmentosa due to monogenic mutation.

Study non-randomized single-group assignment consisting in two sequential cohorts of patients:

- First cohort of two patients with very advanced loss of visual acuity (legally blind)
- Second cohort of ten patients with less advanced loss of visual acuity

Detailed Description
Monocentric study (Hospital of 15–20 at Paris) of duration of 106 weeks.

At total, 12 evaluable patients will be enrolled and assigned in two cohorts as described above in brief summary.

Expected follow-up for one patient is about 64 weeks including 8 weeks of screening and baseline period and 56 weeks of follow-up after implantation of hESC-derived RPE.

After 56 weeks of follow-up, patients will be enrolled in a long-term follow-up study during four additional years.

The primary objective is to assess safety and tolerability of implantation of the Investigational Medicinal Product (ISTEM-01) in patients with retinitis pigmentosa.

Secondary objectives are:

- To evaluate the placement and position of the patch
- To assess preliminary efficacy based on
- Evaluation of visual function
- Eye fundus
- Evaluation of photoreceptor survival

Assessment of visual function by diagnosis-full-field stimulus threshold is the only exploratory objective.

Official Title
A Phase 1/2, Open-Label, Safety, Tolerability, and Preliminary Efficacy Study of Implantation into One Eye of hESC-Derived RPE in Patients with Retinitis Pigmentosa due to Monogenic Mutation

Conditions
Retinitis Pigmentosa

Study Type
Interventional

Enrollment (Actual)
7

Intervention/Treatment
Biological: Human Embryonic Stem Cell Derived Retinal Pigment Epithelium (RPE)

Phase
Phase 1 Phase 2

Study Start (Actual)
2019-08-19

Primary Completion (Estimated)
2023-08-15

Study Completion (Estimated)
2026-12-15

France

Paris, France, 75012
Centre Hospitalier National d'Ophtalmologie (CHNO) des Quinze-Vingts

Eligibility Criteria
Ages Eligible For Study
18–65 years (Adult, Older Adult)

Accepts Healthy Volunteer
No

Sexes Eligible For Study
All

Inclusion Criteria
- Documented diagnosis of retinitis pigmentosa based on a genetic test confirming the presence of a monogenic mutation that affects a gene involved in the visual signaling process specifically at the level of RPEs, namely, RPE65 or LRAT, or MerTK
- 18 years old ≤ Age ≤ 65 years old

  For patient of the first cohort:

- Visual acuity ≤20/200 in the best eye (legally blind)

  For patient of the second cohort:

- 20/63 > Visual acuity >20/200 in the worst eye
- Visible photoreceptor outer nuclear layer (ONL) on a spectral domain OCT scan

For the two cohorts:

- Negative serum pregnancy test in women of childbearing potential (a woman who is 2 year post-menopausal confirmed by a physician or surgically sterile is not considered to be of childbearing potential)
- Female patients of childbearing potential (if sexually active), committed to use two methods of contraception starting from the enrollment, during Mycophenolate Mofetil (MMF) treatment and for 6 weeks after the last dose of MMF
- Sexually active men (including vasectomized men) committed to use condoms during from the first day of MMF treatment and for at least 90 days after cessation of treatment
- Signed informed consents by the patient or legal guardian(s). For patients unable to give consent, authorization to participate to the study will be collected close to their legally authorized representative
- Affiliated to or a beneficiary of a health care system

Exclusion Criteria
- Patient unable or unwilling to comply with the protocol requirements
- History of allergy or sensitivity to one of the products used during the study
- Patients with known serious allergies to the fluorescein
- Patients with a contraindication to general anesthesia
- Prior treatment with a gene or cell therapy product
- Patients with chronic hepatitis B or C, i.e., positive hepatitis B surface antigen or hepatitis CRNA viral load positive
- Patients infected with Human immunodeficiency virus (HIV)
- Anti-HLA antibodies positive at screening
- Pregnancy or breastfeeding
- Presence of any ocular disease or ocular media opacity which in the opinion of the investigator precludes accurate evaluation
- Participation in another drug or device clinical study within last 6 months prior to baseline
- Patients known to be affected by pathologies for which the symptoms or associated treatments can alter the visual function and/or affect the retina
- Systemic corticosteroid therapy or other immunosuppressive/immunomodulating or anti-retroviral drugs within 2 months prior to baseline
- Patients with a contraindication to immunosuppressive/immunomodulating therapy (MMF) such as severe chronic renal impairment, severe digestive system disease, Lesch–Nyhan disease, Kelley–Seegmiller syndrome, etc.
- Acute illness or infection within 4 weeks of the anticipated administration of study medication which may interfere with study assessments and immunosuppressive/immunomodulating therapy
- Any other condition or history that, in the opinion of the Investigator, may compromise the safety or compliance of the patient or would preclude the patient from successful completion of the study

Primary Purpose: Treatment
Allocation: N/A
Interventional Model: Sequential Assignment
Interventional Model Description: Open-label study
Masking: None (Open Label)

Arms and interventions

Participant group/arm	Intervention/treatment
Experimental: Implantation of a therapeutical patch All the patients will receive a single central subretinal implantation in one eye of a monolayer of Human Embryonic Stem Cells-derived Retinal Pigmented Epithelium (hESC-derived RPE). The implanted eye will be the one with the worst visual acuity	Biological: Human Embryonic Stem Cell Derived Retinal Pigment Epithelium (RPE) • Implantation into one eye of hESC-derived RPE [Human Embryonic Stem Cell Derived Retinal Pigment Epithelium (RPE)]

Primary outcome measures

Outcome measure	Measure description	Time frame
Safety assessment	Safety and tolerability measured by the incidence of Adverse Events or Serious Adverse Events throughout the study	From Baseline until week 56

Secondary outcome measures

Outcome measure	Measure description	Time frame
Position of therapeutic patch	Position of the therapeutic patch by serial images assessment	From baseline until week 56
Placement of the therapeutic patch	Placement of the therapeutic patch by serial spectral domain Ocular Coherence Tomography (OCT) scan at baseline and by study visit	From Baseline until week 56
Change in leakage or perfusion	Change in leakage or perfusion in normal fundal vasculature and presence of abnormal vasculature by fundus fluorescein angiography	At baseline and weeks 24, 48, and 56
Change in thickness of RPE layer	Change in thickness of RPE layer by B-mode orbital ultrasound	At weeks 4, 8, 16, 24, 36, 48 and 56

Sponsor
Centre d'Etude des Cellules Souches

Collaborators
No information provided

Investigators
- Principal Investigator: Stéphane BERTIN, MD, Centre des 15-20

General Publications
No publications available

Discussion
This study utilizes hESC-derived RPE. Immunosuppression, with its attendant risks, is required.

Chapter 8
Enrolling by Invitation Stem Cell Studies

United States

Clinical Trial of Autologous Intravitreal Bone-Marrow CD34+ Stem Cells for Retinopathy

ClinicalTrials.gov ID NCT01736059

Sponsor University of California, Davis
Information provided by University of California, Davis (Responsible Party)
Last Update Posted 2022-08-09

Brief Summary
This pilot study is to determine whether it would be safe and feasible to inject CD34+ stem cells from bone marrow into the eye as treatment for patients who are irreversibly blind from various retinal conditions.

Detailed Description
In this pilot clinical trial, eyes with irreversible vision loss from retinal degenerative conditions (macular degeneration or retinitis pigmentosa) or retinal vascular disease (diabetic retinopathy or retinal vein occlusion) will be treated with intravitreal injection of autologous CD34+ stem cells isolated from bone-marrow aspirate under good manufacturing practice conditions. This study will determine whether there are any major safety and feasibility concerns using this therapy. Patients will be followed for 6 months after treatment by serial comprehensive eye examination supplemented with various retinal imaging and diagnostic tests.

Official Title
A Pilot Clinical Trial of the Feasibility and Safety of Intravitreal Autologous Adult Bone-Marrow Stem Cells in Treating Eyes with Vision Loss from Retinopathy.

J. N. Weiss, *Clinical Trials in Retinitis Pigmentosa Treatment*,
https://doi.org/10.1007/978-3-031-58799-3_8

Conditions
Non-exudative Age-related Macular Degeneration
Diabetic Retinopathy
Retina Vein Occlusion
Retinitis Pigmentosa
Hereditary Macular Degeneration

Study Type
Interventional

Enrollment (Estimated)
15

Intervention/Treatment
Drug: CD34+ bone-marrow stem cell intravitreal

Phase
Phase 1

Other Study ID Numbers
906595

Study Start
2012-07

Primary Completion (Estimated)
2023-06

Study Completion (Estimated)
2023-06
United States

Sacramento, California, United States, 95817
University of California Davis

Eligibility Criteria
Ages Eligible For Study
18–100 years (Adult, Older Adult)

Accepts Healthy Volunteer
No

Sexes Eligible for Study
All

Description

Inclusion Criteria
- Age > 18 years of age
- Visual acuity 20/100 to CF
- Duration of vision loss >3 months

- Vision loss from macular degeneration, retinitis pigmentosa, retinal vein occlusion, or diabetic retinopathy
- The study eye has the worse visual acuity
- No active eye or systemic disease
- No history of macular edema or retinal/choroidal neovascularization requiring treatment within 6 months
- No significant media opacity
- No coagulopathy or other hematologic abnormality
- No concurrent immunosuppressive therapy
- Able to keep follow-up for 6 months

Exclusion Criteria

- Allergy to fluorescein dye
- Other concurrent retinal or optic nerve disease affecting vision

Design Details

Primary Purpose: Treatment
Allocation: N/A
Interventional Model: Single Group Assignment
Masking: None (Open Label)

Arms and interventions

Participant group/arm	Intervention/treatment
Experimental: Stem cell treated	Drug: CD34+ bone marrow stem cells intravitreal

Primary outcome measures

Outcome measure	Measure description	Time frame
Incidence and severity of ocular adverse events	As evident on eye examination by severe decrease in vision and/or adverse effect requiring major treatment intervention directly attributable to study treatment	1 day to 6 months

Secondary outcome measures

Outcome measure	Measure description	Time frame
The number of stem cells isolated and injected into the study eye	Will determine the yield of the bone marrow aspiration and stem cell isolation procedures	1 day

Other outcome measures

Outcome measure	Measure description	Time frame
Incidence and severity of systemic adverse events	Any systemic adverse event attributable to the bone marrow aspiration or intravitreal injection of the stem cells	1 day to 6 months

Sponsor

University of California, Davis

Collaborators

No information provided

Investigators

- Principal Investigator: Susanna S Park, MD PhD, University of California Davis Eye Center

General Publications

- Park SS. Cell Therapy Applications for Retinal Vascular Diseases: Diabetic Retinopathy and Retinal Vein Occlusion. Invest Ophthalmol Vis Sci. 2016 Apr 1;57(5):ORSFj1–ORSFj10. https://doi.org/10.1167/iovs.15-17594.

Discussion

As previously discussed, we discontinued intravitreal injection as the results with subtenon/retrobulbar were similar. In addition, patients complained of the opaque floaters, which are even more noticeable when clumped cells are located overlying an area of functional retina. In some cases, it took months for the cells to dissipate.

Enrolling by Invitation

Indonesia

Long-Term Safety of UC-MSC Transplantation in Patients with Retinitis Pigmentosa

ClinicalTrials.gov ID NCT05786287

Sponsor PT. Prodia Stem Cell Indonesia
Information provided by PT. Prodia Stem Cell Indonesia (Responsible Party)
Last Update Posted 2023-06-13

Brief Summary

The study will perform to follow up UC-MSCs and CM transplantation. 18 patients will be called back to be examined after 5 years of UC-MSC and/or CM transplantation.

Detailed Description

The study will be performed on 18 patients who received UC-MSC and CM transplantation in 2018. The study is included as retrospective cohort, since the transplantation happened 5 years ago. Patients will do a visual field test, visual acuity test, electroretinography, funduscopy, and optical coherence tomography examination. The observation results will be written in the observation table and analyzed by a statistic. The study will be performed at Rumah Sakit Jakarta Eye Center and Rumah Sakit Umum Pusat by Dr. Sardjito Yogyakarta.

Official Title

Long-Term Safety of Umbilical Cord-Mesenchymal Stem Cell (UC-MSC) Transplantation in Patients with Retinitis Pigmentosa

Conditions
Retinitis Pigmentosa

Intervention/Treatment
Biological: Conditioned Medium (CM)
Biological: Umbilical Cord-Mesenchymal Stem Cell (UC-MSC)

Study Start (Estimated)
2023-07-01

Primary Completion (Estimated)
2025-07-13

Study Completion (Estimated)
2025-07-13

Enrollment (Estimated)
18

Study Type
Observational

Other Study ID Numbers
CT/RP/08/2022

Indonesia
DKI Jakarta Locations

Jakarta, DKI Jakarta, Indonesia
Jakarta Eye Center Hospital

Special Region Locations
Yogyakarta, Special Region, Indonesia, 55284
Sardjito Hospital

Eligibility Criteria
Inclusion Criteria
- Visual field defects at the initial examination with Humphrey perimetry are between 25% and 50%
- Willing to sign informed consent as research subjects
- Willing to do the peribulbar injection with mesenchymal stem cells isolated from umbilical cord tissue
- Willing to do visual field checks with Humphrey's perimetry, vision tests with Snellen boards, optical coherent tomography (OCT) examinations, electroretinogram examinations and fill out a quality-of-life questionnaire

Exclusion Criteria
- Pregnant or nursing women
- Positive result of HIV test
- Have a history of eye tumors

- In the immunosuppressive treatment or other drugs that can affect the growth of transplanted stem cells
- Have another eye disease such as diabetic retinopathy, uveitis, cataract, and glaucoma
- Do not come to control according to the schedule determined by the researcher (loss to follow up)

Study Population
Retinitis Pigmentosa patients who have been transplanted UC-MSC and/or CM 5 years ago under clinical trials NCT04315025

Ages Eligible for Study
18–65 years (Adult, Older Adult)

Sexes Eligible for Study
All

Accepts Healthy Volunteers
No

Sampling Method
Non-Probability Sample

Design Details
Observational Model: Cohort
Time Perspective: Retrospective

Cohorts and interventions

Group/cohort	Intervention/treatment
Conditioned medium (CM) 2 mL volume of conditioned medium derived umbilical cord Mesenchymal stem cell injected into peribulbar	Biological: Conditioned medium (CM) • Conditioned medium (CM) injected by peribulbar
UC-MSC + NaCl 1.8 mL cell preparations are suspended in physiological NaCl until it reaches a 2 mL volume of cell suspension. Umbilical cord Mesenchymal stem cell (UC-MSC) suspension injected into peribulbar	Biological: Umbilical cord Mesenchymal stem cell (UC-MSC) • Umbilical cord Mesenchymal stem cell (UC-MSC) injected by peribulbar
UC-MSC + CM 1.8 mL cell preparations are suspended in conditioned medium (CM) until it reaches a total of 2 mL volume of cell suspension. Umbilical cord Mesenchymal stem cell (UC-MSC) + conditioned medium (CM) suspension injected into peribulbar	Biological: Conditioned medium (CM) Conditioned medium (CM) injected by peribulbar Biological: Umbilical cord Mesenchymal stem cell (UC-MSC) • Umbilical cord Mesenchymal stem cell (UC-MSC) injected by peribulbar

Primary outcome measures

Outcome measure	Measure description	Time frame
Visual acuity test	a test to see the sharpness of vision using Snellen chart which is read at a distance of 6 m. Normal eye test results are stated in 6/6	5 years after injection
Visual field test	a test to assess the breadth of views of the lateral, medial, superior and inferior aspects using Humprey's perimetry	5 years after injection
Funduscopy	An examination to see and assess the abnormalities and conditions in the ocular fundus using an ophthalmoscope. This examination is carried out by an ophthalmologist	5 years after injection
Electroretinography	An examination to provide a picture of objectivity, a quantitative measure of retinal function to monitor the function of stem cells and ganglion cells in the eye. This examination is carried out by a trained ophthalmologist	5 years after injection
Optical coherence tomography (OCT)	Is a diagnostic test that give the information about posterior segment structure, which is retina and optic nerve papillae so that it can be used to assess macular abnormalities	5 years after injection
Angiography	a process of taking photos of the retina by injecting fluorescent to get a bleeding location on the retina	5 years after injection

Sponsor
PT. Prodia Stem Cell Indonesia

Collaborators
No information provided

Investigators
- Principal Investigator: Dr. Muhammad B Sasongko, Sp. M, M. Epid, PhD, Gadjah Mada University, Faculty of Medicine
- Study Director: Dr. Cosmos O Mangunsong, Sp. M, Jakarta Eye Center
- Study Chair: Dr. Rifa Widyaningrum, M. Sc, PhD, Sardjito Hospital
- Study Chair: Rima Haifa, S. Si, Prodia StemCell Indonesia
- Study Chair: Marsya N Kirana, S.T., M. Sc, Prodia StemCell Indonesia

General Publications
No publications available

Part II
Gene Therapy

Chapter 9
Completed Gene Therapy Studies

United States/Europe

A Clinical Trial of Retinal Gene Therapy for X-Linked Retinitis Pigmentosa Using BIIB112 (XIRIUS)

ClinicalTrials.gov ID NCT03116113

Sponsor NightstaRx Ltd., a Biogen Company
Information provided by NightstaRx Ltd., a Biogen Company (Responsible Party)
Last Update Posted 2023-02-13

Brief Summary
The objective of the study is to evaluate the safety, tolerability, and efficacy of a single sub-retinal injection of BIIB112 in participants with X-linked retinitis pigmentosa (XLRP).

Detailed Description
This study was previously posted by NightstaRx Ltd. In October, 2020, sponsorship of the trial was transferred to Biogen.

Official Title
A Dose Escalation (Phase 1) and Dose Expansion (Phase 2/3) Clinical Trial of Retinal Gene Therapy for X-Linked Retinitis Pigmentosa Using an Adeno-Associated Viral Vector (AAV8) Encoding Retinitis Pigmentosa GTPase Regulator (RPGR)

Conditions
X-Linked Retinitis Pigmentosa

Intervention/Treatment
Biological: BIIB112

J. N. Weiss, *Clinical Trials in Retinitis Pigmentosa Treatment*,
https://doi.org/10.1007/978-3-031-58799-3_9

Study Start (Actual)
2017-03-16

Primary Completion (Actual)
2020-11-18

Study Completion (Actual)
2020-11-18

Enrollment (Actual)
50

Study Type
Interventional

Phase
Phase 1
Phase 2

Other Study ID numbers
274RP101
NSR-RPGR-01 (Other Identifier) (OTHER: NightstaRx Ltd., a Biogen Company)

United States
Florida Locations

Gainesville, Florida, United States, 32607
Research Site

Miami, Florida, United States, 33136
Research Site

Oregon Locations
Portland, Oregon, United States, 97239
Research Site

Pennsylvania Locations

Philadelphia, Pennsylvania, United States, 19104
Research Site

Texas Locations

Dallas, Texas, United States, 75231
Research Site

United Kingdom

Manchester, United Kingdom
Research Site

Oxford, United Kingdom
Research Site

Southampton, United Kingdom
Research Site

Eligibility Criteria
Key Inclusion Criteria
Part 1:
  Participants with genetically confirmed diagnosis of XLRP (with RPGR mutation).
  Participant with active disease clinically visible within the macular region in both eyes.
Part 2:
  Participant with mean total retinal sensitivity in the study eye as assessed by microperimetry ≥0.1 dB and ≤ 8 dB.

Key Exclusion Criteria
Parts 1 and 2:
  Participant with history of amblyopia in either eye.
  Participated in a gene therapy trial previously or a clinical trial with an investigational drug in the past 12 weeks or received a gene/cell-based therapy at any time previously.

Note: Other protocol defined Inclusion/Exclusion criteria may apply.

Ages Eligible for Study
10 years and older (Child, Adult, Older Adult)

Sexes Eligible for Study
Male

Accepts Healthy Volunteers
No

Primary Purpose: Treatment
Allocation: Randomized
Interventional Model: Sequential Assignment
Masking: Quadruple (Participant Care Provider Investigator Outcomes Assessor)

Arms and interventions

Participant group/arm	Intervention/treatment
Experimental: Part 1: BIIB112 dose 1 Participants will receive a single dose 1 of BIIB112 by sub-retinal injection on day 0	Biological: BIIB112 • Administered as specified in the treatment arm • Other names: – AAV8-RPGR
Experimental: Part 1: BIIB112 dose 2 Participants will receive a single dose 2 of BIIB112 by sub-retinal injection on day 0	Biological: BIIB112 • Administered as specified in the treatment arm • Other names: – AAV8-RPGR
Experimental: Part 1: BIIB112 dose 3 Participants will receive a single dose 3 of BIIB112 by sub-retinal injection on day 0	Biological: BIIB112 • Administered as specified in the treatment arm • Other names: – AAV8-RPGR

Experimental: Part 1: BIIB112 dose 4 Participants will receive a single dose 4 of BIIB112 by sub-retinal injection on day 0	Biological: BIIB112 • Administered as specified in the treatment arm • Other names: – AAV8-RPGR
Experimental: Part 1: BIIB112 dose 5 Participants will receive a single dose 5 of BIIB112 by sub-retinal injection on day 0	Biological: BIIB112 • Administered as specified in the treatment arm • Other names: – AAV8-RPGR
Experimental: Part 1: BIIB112 dose 6 Participants will receive a single dose 6 of BIIB112 by sub-retinal injection on day 0	Biological: BIIB112 • Administered as specified in the treatment arm • Other names: – AAV8-RPGR
Experimental: Part 2: BIIB112 high dose Participants will receive a single high dose of BIIB112 by sub-retinal injection	Biological: BIIB112 • Administered as specified in the treatment arm • Other names: – AAV8-RPGR
Experimental: Part 2: BIIB112 low dose Participants will receive a single low dose of BIIB112 by sub-retinal injection	Biological: BIIB112 • Administered as specified in the treatment arm • Other names: – AAV8-RPGR
No intervention: Part 2: Untreated group Participants will receive no intervention to allow for a controlled comparison	

Primary outcome measures

Outcome measure	Measure description	Time frame
Part 1: Number of participants with dose-limiting toxicities (DLTs)	DLTs are defined as any of the following events considered to be related to AAV8-RPGR: Sustained decrease in best-corrected visual acuity (BCVA) of ≥30 letters on the early treatment of diabetic retinopathy study (ETDRS) chart compared to baseline (sustained is defined as lasting 48 h or more until recovery, with recovery defined as visual acuity (VA) returning to within 10 letters of baseline VA. An exception is made for surgery-related events occurring in close temporal association {within <24 h} of the surgery); vitreous inflammation, vitritis (>grade 3 using standardized Nussenblatt vitreous inflammation scale grading); any clinically significant retinal damage observed that is not directly attributed to complications of surgery; any clinically relevant suspected unexpected serious adverse reaction, with the exception of vision loss or vision threatening	Up to month 24
Part 1: Number of participants with treatment-emergent adverse events (TEAEs)	An AE is any untoward medical occurrence in a participant or clinical investigation participant administered a pharmaceutical product and that does not necessarily have a causal relationship with this treatment. An AE can therefore be any unfavorable and unintended sign (including an abnormal laboratory finding), symptom, or disease temporally associated with the use of a medicinal (investigational) product, whether or not related to the medicinal (investigational) product	Up to month 24

Part 2: Percentage of study eyes with ≥7 decibels (dB) improvement from baseline at ≥5 of the 16 central loci of the 10-2 grid assessed by macular integrity assessment (MAIA) Microperimetry	MAIA microperimetry assessment was measured in dB using a 10-2 grid of 68 points. Each point was labeled as '< 0', '0', or a positive integer. The point labeled as '< 0' was assigned a value of '-1' by MAIA in the calculation. Improvement in retinal sensitivity in center grid was defined as an increase from baseline of 7 or more decibels in any 5 or more points out of the 16 central points	Months 12
Part 2: Number of participants with TEAEs	An AE is any untoward medical occurrence in a participant or clinical investigation participant administered a pharmaceutical product and that does not necessarily have a causal relationship with this treatment. An AE can therefore be any unfavorable and unintended sign (including an abnormal laboratory finding), symptom, or disease temporally associated with the use of a medicinal (investigational) product, whether or not related to the medicinal (investigational) product	Up to month 12

Secondary outcome measures

Outcome measure	Measure description	Time frame
Parts 1 and 2: Percentage of study eyes with ≥7 dB improvement from baseline at ≥5 out of the 16 central loci in Microperimetry	MAIA microperimetry assessment was measured in dB using a 10-2 grid of 68 points. Each point was labeled as '< 0', '0' or a positive integer. The point labeled as '< 0' was assigned a value of '-1' by MAIA in the calculation. Improvement in retinal sensitivity in center grid was defined as an increase from baseline of 7 or more decibels in any 5 or more points out of the 16 central points	Part 1: Months 1, 3, 6, 9, 12, 18 and 24; part 2: Months 1, 2, 3, 6, 9, and 12
Parts 1 and 2: Percentage of study eyes with ≥7 dB improvement from baseline at ≥5 out of the 68 loci in Microperimetry	MAIA microperimetry assessment was measured in dB using a 10-2 grid of 68 points. Each point was labeled as '< 0', '0' or a positive integer. The point labeled as '< 0' was assigned a value of '-1' by MAIA in the calculation. Improvement in retinal sensitivity in whole grid was defined as an increase from baseline of 7 or more decibels in any 5 or more points of the grid as a whole (68 points)	Part 1: Months 1, 3, 6, 9, 12, 18 and 24; part 2: Months 1, 2, 3, 6, 9, and 12
Parts 1 and 2: Change from baseline in mean sensitivity of the 16 central loci	MAIA microperimetry assessment was measured in dB using a 10-2 grid of 68 points. Each point was labeled as '< 0', '0' or a positive integer. The point labeled as '< 0' is assigned a value of '-1' by MAIA in the calculation. Improvement in retinal sensitivity in center grid was defined as an increase from baseline of 7 or more decibels in any 5 or more points out of the 16 central points. Here negative values indicate a decline in retinal sensitivity	Part 1: Months 1, 3, 6, 9, 12, 18 and 24; part 2: Months 1, 2, 3, 6, 9, and 12

Outcome measure	Measure description	Time frame
Parts 1 and 2: Change from baseline in mean sensitivity of the 68 central loci	MAIA microperimetry assessment was measured in dB using a 10-2 grid of 68 points. Each point was labeled as '< 0', '0' or a positive integer. The point labeled as '< 0' is assigned a value of '-1' by MAIA in the calculation. Improvement in retinal sensitivity in whole grid was defined as an increase from baseline of 7 or more decibels in any 5 or more points of the grid as a whole (68 points). Here negative values indicate a decline in retinal sensitivity	Part 1: Months 1, 3, 6, 9, 12, 18 and 24; part 2: Months 1, 2, 3, 6, 9, and 12
Parts 1 and 2: Change from baseline in best corrected visual acuity (BCVA) score	BCVA was assessed using the ETDRS VA chart. Initially, letters were read at a distance of 4 m from the chart. If <20 letters were read at 4 m, testing at 1 m was performed. BCVA was to be reported as number of letters read correctly by the subject. An increase in the number of letters read correctly means that vision has improved	Part 1: Months 1, 3, 6, 9, 12, 18 and 24; part 2: Months 1, 2, 3, 6, 9, and 12
Parts 1 and 2: Change from baseline in low luminance visual acuity (LLVA) score	LLVA was measured by placing a 2.0-log-unit neutral density filter over the front of each eye and having the subject read the normally illuminated ETDRS chart. Initially, letters were read at a distance of 4 m from the chart. If <20 letters were read at 4 m, testing at 1 m was performed. LLVA was reported as number of letters read correctly by the subject	Part 1: Months 1, 3, 6, 9, 12, 18, and 24; part 2: Months 1, 3, 6, 9, and 12
Parts 1 and 2: Percentage of eyes with a ≥ 15 letters increase from baseline for BCVA	BCVA was assessed using the ETDRS VA chart. Initially, letters were read at a distance of 4 m from the chart. If <20 letters were read at 4 m, testing at 1 m was performed. BCVA was to be reported as number of letters read correctly by the subject. An increase in the number of letters read correctly means that vision has improved	Part 1: Months 1, 3, 6, 9, 12, 18, and 24; part 2: Months 1, 2, 3, 6, 9, and 12
Parts 1 and 2: Percentage of eyes with a ≥ 15 letters increase from baseline for LLVA	LLVA was measured by placing a 2.0-log-unit neutral density filter over the front of each eye and having the subject read the normally illuminated ETDRS chart. Initially, letters were read at a distance of 4 m from the chart. If <20 letters were read at 4 m, testing at 1 m was performed. LLVA was reported as number of letters read correctly by the subject	Part 1: Months 1, 3, 6, 9, 12, 18, and 24; part 2: Months 1, 3, 6, 9, and 12
Parts 1 and 2: Percentage of eyes with a ≥ 10 letters increase from baseline for BCVA	BCVA was assessed using the ETDRS VA chart. Initially, letters were read at a distance of 4 m from the chart. If <20 letters were read at 4 m, testing at 1 m was performed. BCVA was to be reported as number of letters read correctly by the subject. An increase in the number of letters read correctly means that vision has improved	Part 1: Months 1, 3, 6, 9, 12, 18, and 24; part 2: Months 1, 2, 3, 6, 9, and 12

Outcome measure	Measure description	Time frame
Parts 1 and 2: Percentage of eyes with a ≥ 10 letters increase from baseline for LLVA	LLVA was measured by placing a 2.0-log-unit neutral density filter over the front of each eye and having the subject read the normally illuminated ETDRS chart. Initially, letters were read at a distance of 4 m from the chart. If <20 letters were read at 4 m, testing at 1 m was performed. LLVA was reported as number of letters read correctly by the subject	Part 1: Months 1, 3, 6, 9, 12, 18, and 24; part 2: Months 1, 3, 6, 9, and 12
Parts 1 and 2: Percentage of eyes with a ≥ 5 letters increase from baseline for BCVA	BCVA was assessed using the ETDRS VA chart. Initially, letters were read at a distance of 4 m from the chart. If <20 letters were read at 4 m, testing at 1 m was performed. BCVA was to be reported as number of letters read correctly by the subject. An increase in the number of letters read correctly means that vision has improved	Part 1: Months 1, 3, 6, 9, 12, 18, and 24; part 2: Months 1, 2, 3, 6, 9, and 12
Parts 1 and 2: Percentage of eyes with a ≥ 5 letters increase from baseline for LLVA	LLVA was measured by placing a 2.0-log-unit neutral density filter over the front of each eye and having the subject read the normally illuminated ETDRS chart. Initially, letters were read at a distance of 4 m from the chart. If <20 letters were read at 4 m, testing at 1 m was performed. LLVA was reported as number of letters read correctly by the subject	Part 1: Months 1, 3, 6, 9, 12, 18, and 24; part 2: Months 1, 3, 6, 9, and 12
Parts 1 and 2: Percentage of eyes with a ≥ 15 letters loss from baseline for BCVA	BCVA was assessed using the ETDRS VA chart. Initially, letters were read at a distance of 4 m from the chart. If <20 letters were read at 4 m, testing at 1 m was performed. BCVA was to be reported as number of letters read correctly by the subject. An increase in the number of letters read correctly means that vision has improved	Part 1: Months 1, 3, 6, 9, 12, 18, and 24; part 2: Months 1, 2, 3, 6, 9, and 12
Parts 1 and 2: Percentage of eyes with a ≥ 15 letters loss from baseline for LLVA	LLVA was measured by placing a 2.0-log-unit neutral density filter over the front of each eye and having the subject read the normally illuminated ETDRS chart. Initially, letters were read at a distance of 4 m from the chart. If <20 letters were read at 4 m, testing at 1 m was performed. LLVA was reported as number of letters read correctly by the subject	Part 1: Months 1, 3, 6, 9, 12, 18, and 24; part 2: Months 1, 3, 6, 9, and 12
Parts 1 and 2: Percentage of eyes with a ≥ 10 letters loss from baseline for BCVA	BCVA was assessed using the ETDRS VA chart. Initially, letters were read at a distance of 4 m from the chart. If <20 letters were read at 4 m, testing at 1 m was performed. BCVA was to be reported as number of letters read correctly by the subject. An increase in the number of letters read correctly means that vision has improved	Part 1: Months 1, 3, 6, 9, 12, 18, and 24; part 2: Months 1, 2, 3, 6, 9, and 12

Outcome measure	Measure description	Time frame
Parts 1 and 2: Percentage of eyes with a ≥ 10 letters loss from baseline for LLVA	LLVA was measured by placing a 2.0-log-unit neutral density filter over the front of each eye and having the subject read the normally illuminated ETDRS chart. Initially, letters were read at a distance of 4 m from the chart. If <20 letters were read at 4 m, testing at 1 m was performed. LLVA was reported as number of letters read correctly by the subject	Part 1: Months 1, 3, 6, 9, 12, 18, and 24; part 2: Months 1, 3, 6, 9, and 12
Parts 1 and 2: Percentage of eyes with a ≥ 5 letters loss from baseline for BCVA	BCVA was assessed using the ETDRS VA chart. Initially, letters were read at a distance of 4 m from the chart. If <20 letters were read at 4 m, testing at 1 m was performed. BCVA was to be reported as number of letters read correctly by the subject. An increase in the number of letters read correctly means that vision has improved	Part 1: Months 1, 3, 6, 9, 12, 18, and 24; part 2: Months 1, 2, 3, 6, 9, and 12
Parts 1 and 2: Percentage of eyes with a ≥ 5 letters loss from baseline for LLVA	LLVA was measured by placing a 2.0-log-unit neutral density filter over the front of each eye and having the subject read the normally illuminated ETDRS chart. Initially, letters were read at a distance of 4 m from the chart. If <20 letters were read at 4 m, testing at 1 m was performed. LLVA was reported as number of letters read correctly by the subject	Part 1: Months 1, 3, 6, 9, 12, 18, and 24; part 2: Months 1, 3, 6, 9, and 12
Parts 1 and 2: Percentage of eyes with change from baseline > −5 letters for BCVA	BCVA was assessed using the ETDRS VA chart. Initially, letters were read at a distance of 4 m from the chart. If <20 letters were read at 4 m, testing at 1 m was performed. BCVA was to be reported as number of letters read correctly by the subject. An increase in the number of letters read correctly means that vision has improved	Part 1: Months 1, 3, 6, 9, 12, 18, and 24; part 2: Months 1, 2, 3, 6, 9, and 12
Part 1 and 2: Percentage of eyes with change from baseline > −5 letters for LLVA	LLVA was measured by placing a 2.0-log-unit neutral density filter over the front of each eye and having the subject read the normally illuminated ETDRS chart. Initially, letters were read at a distance of 4 m from the chart. If <20 letters were read at 4 m, testing at 1 m was performed. LLVA was reported as number of letters read correctly by the subject	Part 1: Months 1, 3, 6, 9, 12, 18, and 24; part 2: Months 1, 3, 6, 9, and 12
Part 1: Change from baseline in central ellipsoid area	Spectral domain optical coherence tomography (SD-OCT) was used to assess change in central ellipsoid area	Months 1, 3, 6, 9, 12, 18 and 24
Part 1: Change from baseline in central horizontal ellipsoid width	SD-OCT was used to assess change in central horizontal ellipsoid width. Here negative values indicate decline in central horizontal ellipsoid width	Months 1, 3, 6, 9, 12, 18 and 24
Part 1: Change from baseline in fundus autofluorescence- Total area of preserved autofluorescence	Fundus autofluorescence was used to assess change in total area of preserved autofluorescence and distance from foveal center (FC) to nearest border of preserved autofluorescence	Months 1, 3, 6, 12, 18 and 24

Outcome measure	Measure description	Time frame
Part 1: Change from baseline in fundus autofluorescence-distance from Foveal center (FC) to nearest border of preserved autofluorescence	Fundus autofluorescence was used to assess change in distance from foveal center (FC) to nearest border of preserved autofluorescence	Months 1, 3, 6, 9, 12, 18 and 24
Part 1: Change from baseline in volume of 30-Degree Hill of vision	Visual field testing was performed to assess change in volume of 30-degree hill vision. Reliability factor (RF) = number of false positive responses + number of false negative responses/number of false positive presentations + number of false negative presentations*100. If there are 0 responses, then RF value = 0. RF positive = number of false positive responses/number of false positive presentations*100. If RF ≤ 20% measurement is considered reliable. If 20% < RF ≤ 25% and RF positive ≤10% measurement is also considered reliable. Otherwise, if 20% < RF ≤ 25% and RF positive >10%, or RF > 25%, measurement is not reliable	Months 6, 12 and 24
Part 1: Change from baseline in volume of full Field Hill of vision	Visual field testing was performed to assess change in volume of full field hill vision. Reliability factor (RF) = number of false positive responses + number of false negative responses/number of false positive presentations + number of false negative presentations*100. If there are 0 responses, then RF value = 0. RF positive = number of false positive responses/number of false positive presentations*100. If RF ≤ 20% measurement is considered reliable. If 20% < RF ≤ 25% and RF positive ≤10% measurement is also considered reliable. Otherwise, if 20% < RF ≤ 25% and RF positive >10%, or RF > 25%, measurement is not reliable	Months 6, 12, and 24
Part 1: Change from baseline in contrast sensitivity	Change in contrast sensitivity (CS) was assessed by Pelli-Robson chart which uses a single large letter size (20/60 optotype), with contrast varying across groups of letters. Chart uses letters (6 per line), arranged in groups whose contrast varies from high to low. Subjects read the letters, starting with the highest contrast, until they are unable to read two or three letters in a single group. Each group has three letters of the same contrast level, so there are three trials per contrast level. Subject is assigned a score based on the contrast of the last group in which two or three letters were correctly read. Score is a measure of the subject's log contrast sensitivity ranging from 0 to 2.25, with 0 being no letters read, and 2.25 being all letters read. Total CS score = [(total # letters correct—3) × 0.05]	Months 3, 6, 12 and 24

Outcome measure	Measure description	Time frame
Part 2: Change from baseline in volume of 30-Degree Hill of vision assessed by octopus 900	Visual field testing was performed to assess change in volume of 30-degree hill vision. Reliability factor (RF) = number of false positive responses + number of false negative responses/number of false positive presentations + number of false negative presentations*100. If there are 0 responses, then RF value = 0. RF positive = number of false positive responses/number of false positive presentations*100. If RF ≤ 20% measurement is considered reliable. If 20% < RF ≤ 25% and RF positive ≤10% measurement is also considered reliable. Otherwise, if 20% < RF ≤ 25% and RF positive >10%, or RF > 25%, measurement is not reliable. Here negative values indicate decline in the volume of 30-degree hill vision	Baseline, months 3, 6 and 12
Part 2: Change from baseline in volume of full Field Hill of vision assessed by octopus 900	Visual field testing was performed to assess change in volume of full field hill vision. Reliability factor (RF) = number of false positive responses + number of false negative responses/number of false positive presentations + number of false negative presentations*100. If there are 0 responses, then RF value = 0. RF positive = number of false positive responses/number of false positive presentations*100. If RF ≤ 20% measurement is considered reliable. If 20% < RF ≤ 25% and RF positive ≤10% measurement is also considered reliable. Otherwise, if 20% < RF ≤ 25% and RF positive >10%, or RF > 25%, measurement is not reliable. Here negative values indicate decline in volume of full field hill vision	Baseline, months 3, 6 and 12

Collaborators and Investigators

Sponsor

NightstaRx Ltd., a Biogen Company

Collaborators

No information provided

Investigators

- Study Director: Medical Director, Biogen

General Publications

No publications available

No Results Posted

Completed

United States/Europe

Gene Therapy for X-Linked Retinitis Pigmentosa (XLRP)—Retinitis Pigmentosa GTPase Regulator (RPGR)

ClinicalTrials.gov ID NCT03252847

Sponsor MeiraGTx UK II Ltd.
Information provided by MeiraGTx UK II Ltd. (Responsible Party)
Last Update Posted 2022-12-07

Brief Summary
The Phase 1 part of the study is a dose escalation of subretinal administration of AAV2/5 vector to assess the safety of this vector in participants with XLRP caused by mutations in RPGR.

The Phase 2 part of the study is a cohort expansion of subretinal administration of AAV2/5 vector to assess the safety and efficacy of this vector in participants with XLRP caused by mutations in RPGR.

Detailed Description
This is an open-label phase 1/2 dose-escalation and cohort expansion trial to determine the safety and efficacy of subretinal administration of AAV2/5 vector in participants with XLRP caused by mutations in RPGR.

Official Title
An Open Label, Multi-center, Phase I/II Dose Escalation Trial of a Recombinant Adeno-Associated Virus Vector (AAV2-RPGR) for Gene Therapy of Adults and Children with X-Linked Retinitis Pigmentosa Owing to Defects in Retinitis Pigmentosa GTPase Regulator (RPGR).

Conditions
X-Linked Retinitis Pigmentosa

Intervention/Treatment
Genetic: AAV2/5-RPGR

Study Start (Actual)
2017-07-14

Primary Completion (Actual)
2021-11-18

Study Completion (Actual)
2021-11-18

Enrollment (Actual)
49

Study Type
Interventional

Phase
Phase 1 Phase 2

Other Study ID Numbers
MGT009

Massachusetts Locations

Boston, Massachusetts, United States, 02114
Massachusetts Eye and Ear Institute

Michigan Locations

Ann Arbor, Michigan, United States, 48105
Kellogg Eye Center

Pennsylvania Locations

Pittsburgh, Pennsylvania, United States, 15213
UPMC Eye Center

United Kingdom

Leeds, United Kingdom, LS9 7TF
Leeds Teaching Hospitals NHS Trust

London, United Kingdom
Moorfields Eye Hospital NHS Foundation Trust

Eligibility Criteria
Key Inclusion Criteria
- Are aged 5 years or older male
- Have X-linked retinitis pigmentosa confirmed by a retinal specialist (CI or PI)

Key Exclusion Criteria
- Have participated in another research study involving an investigational medicinal therapy for ocular disease within the last 6 months

Ages Eligible for Study
5 years and older (Child, Adult, Older Adult)

Sexes Eligible for Study
Male

Accepts Healthy Volunteers
No

Primary Purpose: Treatment
Allocation: Randomized
Interventional Model: Sequential Assignment
Interventional Model Description: Biological
Masking: None (Open Label)

Arms and interventions

Participant group/arm	Intervention/treatment
Experimental: Phase 1 (part 1, dose escalation) Participants receive one of three doses of AAV2/5-RPGR	Genetic: AAV2/5-RPGR • Single, subretinal administration of AAV2/5-RPGR
Experimental: Phase 2 (part 2; expansion) Participants receive one of two doses of AAV2/5-RPGR	Genetic: AAV2/5-RPGR • Single, subretinal administration of AAV2/5-RPGR

Primary outcome measures

Outcome measure	Measure description	Time frame
Incidence of adverse events related to the sub retinal administration of AAV2-RPGR	Safety is defined as the absence of advanced therapy medicinal product (ATIMP)-related safety events	18 months

Secondary outcome measures

Outcome measure	Measure description	Time frame
Improvement in visual function	Improvements in visual function as assessed by ocular examination	18 months
Improvement in retinal function	Improvements in retinal function as assessed by retinal assessment	18 months
Improvement in quality of life	• Quality of life will be measured by QoL questionnaire	18 months

Sponsor

MeiraGTx UK II Ltd.

Collaborators

- Syne Qua Non Limited
- Bionical Emas

Investigators

- Principal Investigator: James Bainbridge, Prof, University College, London

General Publications

No publications available

No Results Posted

Completed

United States/Europe

Study to Evaluate Safety and Tolerability of QR-421a in Subjects with RP Due to Mutations in Exon 13 of the USH2A Gene (Stellar)

ClinicalTrials.gov ID NCT03780257

Sponsor ProQR Therapeutics
Information provided by ProQR Therapeutics (Responsible Party)
Last Update Posted 2022-04-20

Brief Summary
The purpose of this study is to evaluate the safety and tolerability of QR-421a administered via intravitreal injection (IVT) in subjects with retinitis pigmentosa (RP) due to mutations in exon 13 of the USH2A gene.

Detailed Description
The purpose of this study is to evaluate the safety and tolerability of QR-421a administered via IVT in subjects with RP due to mutations in exon 13 of the USH2A gene. Subjects will receive one single IVT injection of QR-421a or sham-procedure in one eye (subject's worse eye) and will be followed up for 24 months.

Three dose levels of QR-421a will be evaluated: 50, 100, and 200 μg. Additional dose levels (e.g., 25 or 400 μg) may be evaluated based on ongoing safety and efficacy data monitoring.

Initial dose cohorts will include subjects randomized to sham-procedure or treatment with QR-421a. Additional subjects may be allocated to treatment with QR-421a in subsequent or initial dose cohorts.

Official Title
A First-In-Human Study to Evaluate the Safety and Tolerability of QR-421a in Subjects with Retinitis Pigmentosa (RP) Due to Mutations in Exon 13 of the USH2A Gene

Conditions
Retinitis Pigmentosa
Usher Syndrome Type 2
Deaf Blind
Retinal Disease
Eye Diseases
Eye Diseases, Hereditary
Eye Disorders Congenital
Vision Disorders

Intervention/Treatment
Drug: QR-421a

Other: Sham-procedure (dose cohort 1 and 2 only)

Study Start (Actual)
2019-03-06

Primary Completion (Actual)
2021-10-14

Study Completion (Actual)
2021-10-14

Enrollment (Actual)
20

Study Type
Interventional

Phase
Phase 1 Phase 2

Other Study ID Numbers
PQ-421a-001
2018-002433-38 (EudraCT Number)

United States
Massachusetts Locations

Boston, Massachusetts, United States, 02114
Center for Clinical Research Operations, Massachusetts Eye and Ear

Michigan Locations

Ann Arbor, Michigan, United States, 48105
University of Michigan, Kellogg Eye Center

Oregon Locations

Portland, Oregon, United States, 97239
Casey Eye Institute, Oregon Health & Science University

Texas Locations

Dallas, Texas, United States, 75231
Retina Foundation of the Southwest

Canada

Montréal, Canada, H4A 3 J1
Centre for Innovative Medicine, Department of Pediatric Surgery, Montreal Children's Hospital at the McGill University Health Centre
France

Montpellier, France, 34295
Hôpital Gui de Chauliac-CHRU de Montpellier-Maladies Sensorielles Génétique

Paris, France, 75012
Centre de maladies rares CHNO des Quinze Vingts

Participation Criteria
Researchers look for people who fit a certain description, called eligibility criteria. Some examples of these criteria are a person's general health condition or prior treatments.

Eligibility Criteria
Inclusion Criteria

- Male or female, ≥ 18 years of age.
- Clinical presentation consistent with RP with Usher syndrome type 2 or non-syndromic RP (NSRP), based on ophthalmic, audiologic, and vestibular examinations.
- A molecular diagnosis of homozygosity or compound heterozygosity for 1 or more pathogenic exon 13 mutations in the USH2A gene, based on genetic analysis upon Sponsor approval.
- Impairment of VF in the opinion of the Investigator, as determined by perimetry, with a continuous area of central field greater than or equal to 10 degrees diameter in any axis in the treatment eye, and evidence of functioning rods.
- Willing and able to comply with the protocol, follow study instructions, attend study visits as required and complete all study assessments.
- Willing and able to provide informed consent for participation prior to performing any study related procedures, and suitable verbal, auditory, written and/or tactile sign language communication as to allow informed consent to be obtained, in the opinion of the Investigator.
- No limitations to SD-OCT image collection that would prevent high quality, reliable images from being obtained in both eyes as determined by the investigator.
- Reliable perimetry measurements in both eyes, as described in the Imaging Manual and determined by the Investigator.
- Clear ocular media and adequate pupillary dilation to permit good quality retinal imaging, as assessed by the Investigator.

Exclusion Criteria

- Presence of additional non-exon 13 USH2A pathogenic mutation(s) on the USH2A allele carrying the exon 13 mutation in subjects who are compound heterozygous for mutations in exon 13.
- Presence of non-exon 13 USH2A pathogenic mutation(s) on both USH2A alleles in subjects who are homozygous for mutations in exon 13.
- Presence of pathogenic mutations in genes (other than the USH2A gene) associated with Usher syndrome Type 2 or NSRP, or other inherited retinal degenerative diseases or syndromes.
- Presence of any significant ocular or non-ocular disease/disorder (or medication and/or laboratory test abnormalities) which, in the opinion of the Investigator and with concurrence of the Medical Monitor, may either put the subject at risk because of participation in the study, may influence the results of the study, or the

subject's ability to participate in the study. This includes but is not limited to a subject who: (1) is not an appropriate candidate for antisense oligonucleotide treatment, (2) has cystoid macular edema (CME) in the treatment eye. CME is permissible if stable for 3 months (with or without treatment). Past CME is permissible if resolved for more than 1 month.

- History or presence of ocular herpetic diseases (including herpes simplex virus, varicella zoster or cytomegalovirus) in either eye.
- Presence of any active ocular infection in either eye.
- Presence of any of the following lens opacities in the treatment eye: cortical opacity ≥ +2, posterior subcapsular opacity ≥ +2, or a nuclear sclerosis ≥ +2, and which are: (1) clinically significant in the opinion of the Investigator, (2) would adequately prevent clinical and photographic evaluation of the retina.
- History of amblyopia in the treatment eye.
- Worse than 6 diopters myopia in the treatment eye.
- Receipt within 3 months prior to Screening of any intraocular or periocular surgery (including refractive surgery), or an IVT injection or planned intraocular surgery or procedure during the course of the study.
- Current treatment or treatment within the past 12 months with therapies known to influence the immune system (including but not limited to steroid implants, cytostatics, interferons, tumor necrosis factor (TNF)-binding proteins, drugs acting on immunophilins, or antibodies with known impact on the immune system). Subjects that have been treated with systemic steroids within the past 12 months or that require intermittent use of topical steroids may be considered for inclusion following approval by the Medical Monitor.
- A history of glaucoma or an IOP greater than 24 mmHg in either eye that is not controlled with medication or surgery at the time of informed consent.
- Use of any investigational drug or device within 90 days or 5 half-lives preceding the first dose of study medication, whichever is longer, or plans to participate in another study of an investigational drug or device during the PQ-421a-001 study period.
- Any prior treatment with genetic or stem-cell therapy for ocular or non-ocular disease.
- History of malignancy within 5 years prior to Screening, except adequately treated squamous or basal cell carcinoma of the skin or carcinoma in situ of the cervix that has been successfully treated.
- Known hypersensitivity to antisense oligonucleotides or any constituents of the injection.
- Pregnant and breastfeeding subjects. Females of childbearing potential and males must comply with using highly effective methods of contraception. Women of non-childbearing potential may be included without the use of adequate birth control, provided they meet the criteria in the protocol.

Ages Eligible for Study
18 years and older (Adult, Older Adult)

Sexes Eligible for Study
All

Accepts Healthy Volunteers
No

Design Details
Primary Purpose: Treatment
Allocation: Randomized
Interventional Model: Sequential Assignment
Masking: Quadruple (Participant Care Provider Investigator Outcomes Assessor)

Arms and Interventions

Participant group/arm	Intervention/treatment
Experimental: QR-421a Single dose administration	Drug: QR-421a • RNA antisense oligonucleotide for intravitreal injection • Other names: – RNA antisense oligonucleotide for intravitreal injection
Sham comparator: Sham-procedure (dose cohort 1 & 2 only) Sham-procedure (no experimental drug administered)	Other: Sham-procedure (dose cohort 1 and 2 only) • Sham-procedure (no experimental drug administered) • Other names: – Sham-procedure

Primary outcome measures

Outcome measure	Measure description	Time frame
Incidence and severity of ocular adverse events (AEs) in the treatment and contralateral eye	Incidence and severity of ocular AEs	24 months
Incidence and severity of non-ocular AEs	Incidence and severity of non-ocular AEs	24 months

Secondary outcome measures

Outcome measure	Measure description	Time frame
Change in DAC perimetry	Change in dark adapted chromatic (DAC) perimetry	24 months
Change in static perimetry	Change in static perimetry	24 months
Change in EZ area by SD-OCT	Change in ellipsoid zone (EZ) area/width by spectral domain optical coherence tomography (SD-OCT)	24 months
Change in BCVA	Change in best corrected visual acuity (BCVA)	24 months
Change in LLVA	Change in low luminance visual acuity (LLVA)	24 months
Change in microperimetry	Change in microperimetry	24 months
Changes in FST	Changes in full-field stimulus threshold (FST)	24 months
Changes in FAF	Changes in fundus autofluorescence (FAF)	24 months
AUC (0–∞) of QR-421a in serum	Area under the curve 0 h to infinity [AUC(0–∞)] of QR-421a in serum	24 months

AUC (0-tlast) of QR-421a in serum	Area under the curve 0 h to the final sample with a concentration greater than lower limit of quantification (LLOQ) [AUC(0-tlast)] of QR-421a in serum	24 months
Cmax of QR-421a in serum	Maximum concentration (Cmax) of QR-421a in serum	24 months
Tmax of QR-421a	Time to maximum concentration (Tmax) of QR-421a	24 months
T1/2 of QR-421a	Terminal elimination half-life (T1/2) of QR-421a	24 months
Serum clearance (CL) of QR-421a	Serum clearance (CL) of QR-421a	24 months
Volume of distribution (Vd) of QR-421a	Volume of distribution (Vd) of QR-421a	24 months

Sponsor
ProQR Therapeutics

Collaborators
No information provided

Investigators
- Study Director: ProQR Medical Monitor, ProQR Therapeutics
- Study Director: ProQR Clinical Trial Manager, ProQR Therapeutics

General Publications
No publications available

Results submitted—quality control review has not concluded

Completed

India

Dose-Escalation Study to Evaluate the Safety and Tolerability of Intravitreal vMCO-I in Patients with Advanced Retinitis Pigmentosa

ClinicalTrials.gov ID NCT04919473

Sponsor Nanoscope Therapeutics Inc.
Information provided by Nanoscope Therapeutics Inc. (Responsible Party)
Last Update Posted 2021-06-09

Brief Summary
The purpose of the study is to evaluate the safety and tolerability of a single intravitreal injection of virally-carried Multi-Characteristic Opsin I (vMCO-I).

Detailed Description
This open label dose-escalation study evaluated two dose levels in up to 11 subjects of retinitis pigmentosa (three in low dose and eight in high dose per dose) with

active vMCO-010. Subjects with confirmed diagnosis of Advanced Retinitis Pigmentosa (RP) based on clinical examination and dilated fundus examination, were considered for participation in this study. The primary endpoint for this study is safety and tolerability of vMCO-I at 16 weeks. All subjects were assessed for 52 weeks following treatment with vMCO-I.

Official Title
A Phase I/IIa Open Label, Dose-Escalation Study to Evaluate the Safety and Tolerability of Intravitreal vMCO-I in Patients with Advanced Retinitis Pigmentosa.

Conditions
Retinitis Pigmentosa
Retinal Diseases
Retinal Degeneration

Intervention/Treatment
Biological: Gene Therapy product: vMCO-I

Study Start (Actual)
2019-10-23

Primary Completion (Actual)
2020-02-25

Study Completion (Actual)
2020-10-31

Enrollment (Actual)
11

Study Type
Interventional

Phase
Phase 1 Phase 2

Other Study ID Numbers
NSCT/CT/18/01

India
Odisha Locations

Cuttack, Odisha, India, 753014
JPM Rotary Club of Cuttack Eye Hospital and Research Institute

Eligibility Criteria
Inclusion Criteria
- Age > 18 years
- Diagnosis of advanced RP using Fundus Photographs
- Clinical diagnosis of advanced retinal dystrophy

- Prior documented (if any) retinal electrophysiological evidence of rod-cone photoreceptor degeneration
- Snellen's visual acuity equivalent LP/NLP in worse (study) eye
- Visual acuity in the non-study eye of no-better-than finger counting
- Presence of retinal bipolar cells and retinal nerve fiber layer on OCT testing

Exclusion Criteria

- Prior participation in a clinical study (ocular or non-ocular) with an investigational drug, agent or therapy or any gene or stem cell therapy in the past 6 months.
- Concurrent participation in another interventional clinical ocular study.
- Pre-existing eye conditions such as glaucoma, diseases affecting the optic nerve causing significant visual field loss, active uveitis, corneal or lenticular opacities).
- Presence of any complicating systemic diseases such as malignancies whose treatment could affect central nervous system function.
- Subjects who are positive for hepatitis B, C, and HIV will be excluded.
- Subjects who have undergone ocular surgery in the study eye within 3 months prior to day 0.
- Presence of narrow iridocorneal angles contraindicating pupillary dilation in the study eye.
- Known sensitivity to any component of the study agent or medications planned for use in the peri-operative period.
- Subjects will be excluded if immunological studies show presence of neutralizing antibodies to AAV2 above 1:1000.
- Presence of narrow iridocorneal angles contraindicating pupillary dilation.
- Presence of disorders of the ocular media which interfere with visual acuity and other ocular assessments, including OCT, during the study period.
- Presence of vitreo-macular adhesion or traction, epiretinal membrane, macular pucker and macular hole, evident by ophthalmoscopy and/or by OCT examinations and assessed by the investigator to significantly affect central vision.
- Current evidence of retinal detachment assessed by the investigator to significantly affect central vision.
- Active ocular inflammation or recurrent history of idiopathic or autoimmune-associated uveitis.

Ages Eligible for Study
18 years and older (Adult, Older Adult)

Sexes Eligible for Study
All

Accepts Healthy Volunteers
No

Design Details
Primary Purpose: Treatment
Allocation: Non-Randomized
Interventional Model: Sequential Assignment
Masking: None (Open Label)

Arms and interventions

Participant group/arm	Intervention/treatment
Experimental: vMCO-I high dose Participants received 3.5E11vg/ eye of vMCO-I	Biological: Gene therapy product: vMCO-I • The vMCO-I is an adeno-associated virus serotype 2-based vector carried multi-characteristic opsin (MCO) gene expression cassette
Experimental: vMCO-I low dose Participants received 1.75E11vg/ eye of vMCO-I	Biological: Gene therapy product: vMCO-I • The vMCO-I is an adeno-associated virus serotype 2-based vector carried multi-characteristic opsin (MCO) gene expression cassette

Primary outcome measures

Outcome measure	Measure description	Time frame
The safety and tolerability of escalating doses of vMCO-1 administered via a single IVT in subjects with advanced retinitis Pigmentosa	Safety and tolerability of vMCO-1 treatment at week 16, by assessments based on local and systemic safety issues, as assessed by incidence of adverse events	16 weeks

Secondary outcome measures

Outcome measure	Measure description	Time frame
Evaluate the treatment effect of vMCO-1 as assessed by visual acuity	Assessment of the treatment effect with the change from baseline to week 52 of parameters measured with the Freiburg visual acuity (FrACT) to provide automated, self-paced, monitored measurement	52 weeks
Evaluate the treatment effect of vMCO-1 as assessed by visually-guided mobility assays	Assessment of the treatment effect with the change from baseline to week 52 of parameters measured with light-guided mobility assays, performed at different light intensities, to provide functional vision measures using the time to find lighted panel	52 weeks
Evaluate the treatment effect of vMCO-1 as assessed by visually-guided mobility assays	Assessment of the treatment effect with the change from baseline to week 52 of parameters measured with light-guided mobility assays, performed at different light intensities, to provide functional vision measures using the score based on correct choice	52 weeks
Evaluate the treatment effect of vMCO-1 as assessed by static shape recognition assay	Assessment of the treatment effect with the change from baseline to week 52 of parameters measured with static shape recognition assay, performed at different light intensities, to provide visual function measures using size determination threshold	52 weeks
Evaluate the treatment effect of vMCO-1 as assessed by static shape recognition assay	Assessment of the treatment effect with the change from baseline to week 52 of parameters measured with static shape recognition assay, performed at different light intensities, to provide visual function measures using % shape recognition accuracy	52 weeks
Evaluate the treatment effect of vMCO-1 as assessed by optical flow assay	Assessment of the treatment effect with the change from baseline to week 52 of parameters measured with optical flow assay, performed at different speeds, to provide visual function measures using the %accuracy in determining direction of flow	52 weeks

Evaluate the treatment effect of vMCO-1 as assessed by optical flow assay	Assessment of the treatment effect with the change from baseline to week 52 of parameters measured with optical flow assay, performed at different speeds, to provide visual function measures using the upper speed limit to determine correct optical flow	52 weeks
Evaluate the treatment effect of vMCO-1 as assessed by quality of life questionnaire	Assessment of the treatment effect on quality of life changes from baseline to week 52 with visual function Questionnaire-25 (VFQ-25). VFQ25 is a 25-item questionnaire with 47 questions, each question has several responses scored on a scale from 0-5, 0-6, or 0-10. Values are calculated in percentages.	52 weeks
Evaluate the treatment effect of vMCO-1 as assessed by Humphrey visual field	Assessment of the treatment effect with the change from baseline to week 52 with Humphrey visual field (30-2). Visual field index (VFI) is calculated in % and mean deviation (MD) values are calculated in dB	52 weeks

Sponsor
Nanoscope Therapeutics Inc.

Collaborators
No information provided

Investigators
- Principal Investigator: Santosh Mahapatra, MD, JPM Rotary Club of Cuttack Eye Hospital and Research Institute

General Publications
No publications available

No Results Posted

Completed

Saudi Arabia

Trial of Subretinal Injection of (rAAV2-VMD2-hMERTK)

ClinicalTrials.gov ID NCT01482195

Sponsor King Khaled Eye Specialist Hospital
Information provided by King Khaled Eye Specialist Hospital (Responsible Party)
Last Update Posted 2022-01-26

Brief Summary
This study was to assess the safety of gene transfer via subretinal administration of rAAV2-VMD2-hMERTK in subjects with MERTK-associated retinitis pigmentosa (RP).

Detailed Description

In this phase I open-label, dose-escalation trial, one eye of each patient (the worse-seeing eye in five subjects) will receive a submacular injection of the subretinal rAAV2–VMD2–hMERTK. Patients will be followed daily for 10 days and then at 30, 60, 90, 180, 270, 365, 540, and 730 day post-injection. Data will be collected on (1) full ophthalmologic examination including best-corrected VA, intraocular pressure, color fundus photographs, macular spectral-domain optical coherence tomography, and full-field stimulus threshold test (FST) in both the study and fellow eyes; (2) systemic safety data including CBC, liver, and kidney function tests, coagulation profiles, urine analysis, AAV antibody titers, peripheral blood PCR and ASR measurement; and (3) listing of ophthalmological or systemic adverse effects.

Official Title

Phase I Trial of Ocular Subretinal Injection of a Recombinant Adeno-Associated Virus (rAAV2-VMD2-hMERTK) Gene Vector to Patients with Retinal Disease Due to MERTK Mutations

Conditions

Retinal Disease
Retinitis Pigmentosa

Intervention/Treatment

Biological: Subretinal administration of rAAV2-VMD2-hMERTKRecombinant Adeno-Associated Virus

Study Start (Actual)

2011-08

Primary Completion (Actual)

2013-08

Study Completion (Actual)

2019-08

Enrollment (Actual)

6

Study Type

Interventional

Phase

Phase 1

Other Study ID Numbers

0916-P

Contacts and Locations
Saudi Arabia

Riyadh, Saudi Arabia, 11462
King Khaled Eye Specialist Hospital

Eligibility Criteria

Inclusion Criteria

- MERTK-associated retinal disease;
- VA: 20/100 or less in worse eye
- Ability to perform tests of visual and retinal function;
- Good general health based on a complete physical examination and hematology and chemistry studies performed at a pre-treatment evaluation;
- Ability to comply with research procedures;

Exclusion Criteria

- Pre-existing eye conditions that would preclude the planned surgery or interfere with the interpretation of study endpoints or surgical complications (for example, glaucoma, corneal, or lenticular opacities);
- Complicating systemic diseases (such as medical conditions causing immunosuppression) that would preclude the gene transfer, ocular surgery or known sensitivity or allergy to medications planned for use in the peri-operative period;
- Use of anti-platelet agents that may alter coagulation within 7 days prior to study agent administration;
- Use of immunosuppressive medications;
- Pregnancy or breastfeeding;
- Individuals (males and females) of childbearing potential who are unwilling to use effective contraception for 1 year following agent administration and barrier contraception for 3 months following agent administration;
- Any other condition that would prevent a subject from completing follow-up examinations during the course of the study and that, in the opinion of the investigator, makes the subject unsuitable for the study.
- Current, or recent (within the past 30 days, or 10 half-lives of the drug) participation, in any other research protocol involving investigational agents or therapies.
- Recent (within past 6 months) receipt of an investigational biologic therapeutic agent. Subjects will not be excluded based on their gender, race, or ethnicity.

Ages Eligible for Study

14–70 years (Child, Adult, Older Adult)

Sexes Eligible for Study

All

Accepts Healthy Volunteers

No

Design Details

Primary Purpose: Treatment
Allocation: Non-Randomized
Interventional Model: Single Group Assignment
Interventional Model Description: Ocular Subretinal administration of rAAV2-VMD2-hMERTK.
Masking: None (Open Label)

Arms and interventions

Participant group/arm	Intervention/treatment
Experimental: Subretinal injection of rAAV2-VMD2-hMERTKRecombinant Adeno-associated virus Single arm of 6 patients undergoing subretinal injection of gene therapy using rAAV2-VMD2-hMERTKRecombinant Adeno-associated virus. Each patient received the injection in one eye	Biological: Subretinal administration of rAAV2-VMD2-hMERTKRecombinant Adeno-associated virus • The study is an open-label, dose-escalation, phase I clinical trial of subretinal administration of rAAV2-VMD2-hMERTK in patients with retinitis pigmentosa due to MERTK mutation
No intervention: Fellow eye without intervention Fellow eye without intervention	

Primary outcome measures

Outcome measure	Measure description	Time frame
Systemic and ocular safety	Detailed history & physical exam were obtained at baseline visit and each post-injection protocol visit searching for systemic adverse events. Included were electrocardiogram, chest X-ray, complete blood count & differential, prothrombin time & INR, partial thromboplastin time, serum electrolytes, full serum chemistries including liver and renal function, urinalysis; serum antibody titers to AAV2 capsid components and antigen-specific reactivity (ASR) assays; blood analysis by DNA PCR to detect vector spread Ophthalmic safety monitored changes from baseline included (1) corneal abnormalities, afferent pupillary defect, intraocular inflammation, cataract & intraocular pressure changes; (2) retinal changes based on fundus photos; (3) macular SD-OCT changes in central macular (CMT) and central foveal thickness (CFT) measurements when patient fixation allowed it, and (4) full field stimulus threshold (FST) to detect any retinal toxicity	2 years

Secondary outcome measures

Outcome measure	Measure description	Time frame
Visual acuity measurement	Although candidates may have very severe loss of function, an attempt was made to measure a best-corrected visual acuity using Early Treatment Diabetic Retinopathy Study (ETDRS) charts, and measurements were recorded as the number of letters read on each line of the chart (Diabetic Retinopathy Study Research Group 1985). If a patient was unable to read at least three letters of the first line correctly, the chart distance was progressively halved from the standard 4 m until either the first line was correctly read or the shortest distance of 0.5 m was reached. Patients who were unable to read any letters on the chart were tested for light perception and if they perceived light, they were assigned the acuity score equivalent of <20/6400. Measurements were performed at baseline and each protocol follow up visit. Improvement in patients who could read was defined as a gain in 5 letters, and in those with those LP vision only to start seeing hand motion	2 years and up to 5 years

Full-field stimulus threshold testing (FST)	Full-field stimulus threshold testing (FST) measures sensitivity of the entire visual field by estimating the lowest luminance of a flash that elicits a visual sensation. The FST measurements were performed at baseline and throughout the protocol visits over 2 years in the study and fellow eyes, and changes in FST results were analyzed	2 years
Central Foveal thickness (CFT) on optical coherence tomography (OCT)	Central foveal thickness (CFT) measurements were performed at baseline and throughout the protocol visits over 2 years in the study and fellow eyes (whenever possible), and changes in CFT values were analyzed	2 years
Central macular thickness (CMT) on optical coherence tomography (OCT)	Central macular thickness (CMT) measurements were performed at baseline and throughout the protocol visits over 2 years in the study and fellow eyes (whenever possible), and changes in CMT values were analyzed	2 years

Collaborators and Investigators

This is where you will find people and organizations involved with this study.

Sponsor

King Khaled Eye Specialist Hospital

Collaborators

- King Faisal Specialist Hospital & Research Center

Investigators

- Principal Investigator: Fowzan S Alkuraya, MD, King Faisal Specialist Hospital & Research Center

General Publications

No publications available

Results

Outcomes and adverse events

1. Systemic and ocular safety

Type: Primary|Time Frame: 2 years

Description	Detailed history and physical exam were obtained at baseline visit and each post-injection protocol visit searching for systemic adverse events. Included were electrocardiogram, chest X-ray, complete blood count & differential, prothrombin time & INR, partial thromboplastin time, serum electrolytes, full serum chemistries including liver and renal function, urinalysis; serum antibody titers to AAV2 capsid components and antigen-specific reactivity (ASR) assays; blood analysis by DNA PCR to detect vector spread Ophthalmic safety monitored changes from baseline included (1) corneal abnormalities, afferent pupillary defect, intraocular inflammation, cataract & intraocular pressure changes; (2) retinal changes based on fundus photos; (3) Macular SD-OCT changes in Central macular (CMT) and central foveal thickness (CFT) measurements when patient fixation allowed it, and (4) full field stimulus threshold (FST) to detect any retinal toxicity
Time frame	2 years
Analysis population description	[not specified]

Arm/group title	Recombinant adeno-associated virus injected eyes	Fellow eyes
Arm/group description	Eyes with RP which received a single dose of subretinal recombinant Adeno-associated virus injection	Eyes with RP which did not receive subretinal recombinant Adeno-associated virus injection
Overall number of participants analyzed	6	6
Systemic events [a]measure type: Count of participants|unit of measure: Participants	00.0%	00.0%
Corneal abnormalities[a]	116.7%	00.0%
Afferent pupillary defect[a]	00.0%	00.0%
Intraocular inflammation[a]	00.0%	00.0%
Cataract[a]	116.7%	00.0%
Intraocular pressure changes[a]	00.0%	00.0%
Retinal changes[a]	233.3%	233.3%
Macular thinning on OCT[a]	00.0%	116.7%
Toxicity seen on FST[a]	00.0%	00.0%

[a] Measure type: Count of participants|unit of measure: Participants

2. Visual acuity measurement

Type: Secondary|Time Frame: 2 years and up to 5 years

Description	Although candidates may have very severe loss of function, an attempt was made to measure a best-corrected visual acuity using Early Treatment Diabetic Retinopathy Study (ETDRS) charts, and measurements were recorded as the number of letters read on each line of the chart (Diabetic Retinopathy Study Research Group 1985). If a patient was unable to read at least three letters of the first line correctly, the chart distance was progressively halved from the standard 4 m until either the first line was correctly read or the shortest distance of 0.5 m was reached. Patients who were unable to read any letters on the chart were tested for light perception, and if they perceived light, they were assigned the acuity score equivalent of <20/6400. Measurements were performed at baseline and each protocol follow up visit. Improvement in patients who could read was defined as a gain in five letters, and in those with those LP vision only to start seeing hand motion
Time frame	2 years and up to 5 years
Analysis population description	[not specified]

Arm/group title	Recombinant adeno-associated virus injected eyes	Fellow eyes
Arm/group description	Eyes with RP which received a single dose of subretinal recombinant Adeno-associated virus injection	Eyes with RP which did not receive subretinal recombinant Adeno-associated virus injection
Overall number of participants analyzed	6	6
Improved VA at 2 years [a]measure type: Count of participants|unit of measure: Participants	350.0%	116.7%
Decreased VA at 2 years[a]	00.0%	233.3%
Stable VA at 2 years[a]	350.0%	350.0%
Improvement of VA after 2 years[a]	00.0%	00.0%

[a] Measure type: Count of participants|unit of measure: Participants

3. Full-field stimulus threshold testing (FST)

Type: Secondary|Time Frame: 2 years

Description	Full-field stimulus threshold testing (FST) measures sensitivity of the entire visual field by estimating the lowest luminance of a flash that elicits a visual sensation. The FST measurements were performed at baseline and throughout the protocol visits over 2 years in the study and fellow eyes, and changes in FST results were analyzed.
Time frame	2 years
Analysis population description	Six patients with the clinical diagnosis of RP with a proven MERTK mutation were included. Patients had to be older than 14 years of age and had the viral vector injected into their worse seeing one eye (except case #4)

Arm/group title	Recombinant adeno-associated virus injected eyes	Fellow eyes
Arm/group description	Eyes with RP which received a single dose of subretinal recombinant Adeno-associated virus injection	Eyes with RP which did not receive subretinal recombinant Adeno-associated virus injection
Overall number of participants analyzed	6	6
FST at baseline		
Number analyzed	6 participants	6 participants
[a]mean (95% confidence interval)|unit of measure: dB	−23.34(−29.65 to −17.03)	−24.14(−30.40 to −17.88)
FST at 10 days		
Number analyzed	6 participants	6 participants
[a]	−19.58(−25.93 to −13.23)	−20.13(−26.59 to −13.67)
FST at 30 days		
Number analyzed	6 participants	6 participants
[a]	−19.22(−23.98 to −14.46)	−23.40(−30.60 to −16.29)
FST at 90 days		
Number analyzed	5 participants	6 participants
[a]	−13.94(−42.96 to 15.08)	−24.68(−33.54 to −15.82)
FST at 180 days		
Number analyzed	4 participants	6 participants
[a]	−20.01(−28.12 to −11.90)	−22.02(−31.83 to −12.21)
FST at 365 days		
Number analyzed	5 participants	6 participants
[a]	−20.59(−30.09 to −11.08)	−22.26(−28.87 to −15.65)
FST at 1.5 year		
Number analyzed	5 participants	6 participants
[a]	−21.09(−29.04 to −13.14)	−21.66(−29.81 to −13.51)
FST at 2 years		
Number analyzed	3 participants	6 participants
[a]	−20.38(−28.54 to −12.23)	−15.92(−29.78 to −2.05)

[a] Mean (95% confidence interval)|unit of measure: dB

4. Central foveal thickness (CFT) on optical coherence tomography (OCT)

Type: Secondary|Time Frame: 2 years

Description	Central foveal thickness (CFT) measurements were performed at baseline and throughout the protocol visits over 2 years in the study and fellow eyes (whenever possible), and changes in CFT values were analyzed
Time frame	2 years
Analysis population description	[not specified]

Arm/group title	Recombinant adeno-associated virus injected eyes	Fellow eyes
Arm/group description	Eyes with RP which received a single dose of subretinal recombinant Adeno-associated virus injection	Eyes with RP which did not receive subretinal recombinant Adeno-associated virus injection
Overall number of participants analyzed	5	5
CFT at baseline [a]mean (95% confidence interval)|unit of measure: Microns	65.80 (36.69–94.91)	74.80 (41.22–108.38)
CFT at 2 years[a]	69.20 (39.89–98.51)	75.00 (50.51–99.49)

[a] Mean (95% confidence interval)|unit of measure: Microns

5. Central macular Thickness (CMT) on optical coherence tomography (OCT)

Type: Secondary|Time Frame: 2 years

Description	Central macular thickness (CMT) measurements were performed at baseline and throughout the protocol visits over 2 years in the study and fellow eyes (whenever possible), and changes in CMT values were analyzed
Time frame	2 years
Analysis population description	[not specified]

Arm/group title	Recombinant adeno-associated virus injected eyes	Fellow eyes
Arm/group description	Eyes with RP which received a single dose of subretinal recombinant Adeno-associated virus injection	Eyes with RP which did not receive subretinal recombinant Adeno-associated virus injection
Overall number of participants analyzed	3	3
CMT at baseline [a]mean (95% confidence interval)|unit of measure: Microns	128.00 (65.75–190.25)	132.67 (40.56–224.76)
CMT at 2 years[a]	132.33 (70.76–193.90)	123.76 (48.92–198.41)

[a] Mean (95% confidence interval)|unit of measure: Microns

Adverse Event Reporting Description

The adverse events were collected:

1. Systematically (blood samples withdrawn to test for rise in anti-viral titers). One temporary rise occurred in the post-operative period in one patient = non serious adverse events)
2. Nonsystematic collection: (one patient reported filamentary keratitis, another patient reported oscillopsia in the injected eye- = Other non-serious adverse events

Arm/group title	Recombinant adeno-associated virus	
Arm/group description	Recombinant Adeno-associated virus: Ocular subretinal injection of a recombinant Adeno-associated virus	
All-cause mortality		
Arm/group Title	Recombinant Adeno-associated virus	
	Affected/at risk (%)	
Total	0/6 (0.00%)	
Serious adverse events		
Arm/group Title	Recombinant Adeno-associated virus	
	Affected/at risk (%)	# events
Total	0/6 (0.00%)	
Other (not including serious) adverse events		
0% Frequency threshold for reporting other adverse events		
Arm/group Title	Recombinant Adeno-associated virus	
	Affected/at risk (%)	# events
Total	3/6 (50.00%)	
Blood and lymphatic system disorders		
Systemic [a, b]	1/6 (16.67%)	1
Eye disorders		
Filamentary keratitis[a, c]	1/6 (16.67%)	1
Delayed resolution of subretinal fluid postoperatively, cataract, oscillopsia[a, d]	1/6 (16.67%)	1

[a] Indicates events were collected by systematic assessment

[b] One patient developed a rise in AAV antibodies but with a negative PCR. Serum AAV antibody and antigen specific reactivity measurements for the remaining patients are negative

[c] Resolved with postoperative lubrication therapy

[d] The fluid resolved spontaneously within 6 weeks after surgery with return of vision to baseline. The same patient developed posterior subcapsular cataract and persistent oscillopsia in the operated eye and the cause remains unknown

Chapter 10
Active, Recruiting Gene Therapy Studies

United States/Europe

Promising ROd-Cone DYstrophy Gene therapY (PRODYGY)

ClinicalTrials.gov ID NCT05748873

Sponsor SparingVision
Information provided by SparingVision (Responsible Party)
Last Update Posted 2023-06-01

Brief Summary
This is a two-step, multicenter, phase I/II study including an open-label dose-escalation phase (Step 1) and a three-arm controlled double-masked randomized extension phase (Step 2), in subjects with advanced RCD due to a mutation in the RHO, PDE6A, or PDE6B gene.

Official Title
A Phase I/II Study to Assess the Safety and Tolerability of a Single Subretinal Administration of SPVN06 Gene Therapy in Subjects with Rod-Cone Dystrophy (RCD) due to a Mutation in the RHO, PDE6A, or PDE6B Gene

Conditions
Retinitis pigmentosa

Intervention/Treatment
Drug: SPVN06

Study Start (Actual)
2023-04-12

Primary Completion (Estimated)
2025-03

J. N. Weiss, *Clinical Trials in Retinitis Pigmentosa Treatment*,
https://doi.org/10.1007/978-3-031-58799-3_10

Study Completion (Estimated)
2029-03

Enrollment (Estimated)
33

Study Type
Interventional

Phase
Phase 1 Phase 2

Other Study ID Numbers
SPVN06-CLIN-01

Study Contact
Name: SparingVision
Phone number: +33143462060
Email: info@sparingvision.com

Study Contact Backup
Name: Medical Director
United States
Pennsylvania locations

Pittsburgh, Pennsylvania, United States, 15213
Recruiting
UPMC Eye Center

Contact
Natalie Anthony
412-647-5756 anthonynl2@upmc.edu

Contact
Rhonda Dahlstrom
412-647-5756 dahlstromrj@upmc.edu
Principal Investigator:
Joseph Martel, MD

France

Paris, France, 75012
Recruiting
CHNO XV-XX Paris—CIC 1423

Contact
Berthe Pom
+33635230695 bpom@15-20.fr
Principal Investigator:
Isabelle Audo, MD, PhD

Inclusion Criteria

Subjects will be eligible to participate in this study only if all the following criteria apply:

- Able to give signed informed consent and comply with the requirements and restrictions listed in the informed consent form (ICF) and in the protocol.
- Age ≥ 18 years at the time of ICF signature.
- Subjects of either gender previously diagnosed with advanced RCD due to biallelic mutations in the rod cGMP phosphodiesterase 6 beta (PDE6B) or rod cGMP phosphodiesterase alpha (PDE6A) genes, or due to a monoallelic dominant mutation in the rhodopsin (RHO) gene. The genotyping results must be documented before the initiation of the Screening Visit. Subjects should be retested by the investigator if their genotyping tests were not performed within the 3 previous years, or if they were not performed by an accredited laboratory. In this case, the screening period can be prolonged for 2 additional weeks to allow time to generate genotyping results.
- Advanced stage is defined as a stage of the natural history of the disease where both distance visual acuity and visual field are affected in both eyes. Substages within the advanced stage are defined as follows (monocular measurements, horizontal axis of isopter III4e for the visual field):
  - Severe stage is defined by both a BCVA below or equal to 20/200 and above or equal to 20/400, and a visual field below or equal to 20 degrees (subjects of Cohorts 1–3)
  - Intermediate stage is defined by both a BCVA below or equal to 20/40 and above 20/200, and a visual field below or equal to 20 degrees (subjects of Cohorts 4–6)
- Regardless of the severity of the disease, the difference in visual acuity between the two eyes of a given subject should be equal to or below 0.3 logarithm of the minimal angle (LogMAR) (≤ 3 ETDRS lines)
- Clinical diagnosis of RCD based on past medical and family history, midperipheral visual field dysfunction, photopsia, night blindness (nyctalopia), and fundoscopic appearance (including but not restricted to bone spicule pigmentation, attenuation of the retinal vessels, and waxy pallor of the optic nerve).
- Diagnosis of RCD is confirmed on prior full-field ERG (any previously performed ERG is acceptable).
- Documented preservation of cone inner and outer segments considered good enough by the investigator for the subject to be included in the study.
- Negative serum pregnancy test for women of childbearing potential (please refer to Schedule of Assessments for details).
- Women of childbearing potential (WOCBP) and men and/or their partner(s) of childbearing potential must agree to use a highly effective contraceptive method. This applies to the time period between ICF signature and 12 months after SPVN06 SRI. The definition of highly effective contraceptive methods follows CTFG recommendations. Highly effective contraceptive methods are limited to:

- Combined (estrogen and progestogen containing) hormonal contraception associated with inhibition of ovulation:

  Oral
  Intravaginal
  Transdermal

- Progestogen-only hormonal contraception associated with inhibition of ovulation:
  Oral
  Injectable
  Implantable

- Intrauterine device (IUD)
- Intrauterine hormone-releasing system (IUS)
- Bilateral tubal occlusion
- Vasectomized partner
- Sexual abstinence

• Subjects must be affiliated to a health security system, if they are included in a clinical site based in France (per law).
• No out-of-range values for clinical laboratory tests; however, if outside, it must be considered as nonclinically relevant by the investigator using a multidisciplinary approach and compatible with a participation in the clinical study.
• A 12-lead electrocardiogram within normal limits, however, when outside, must be documented by the investigator using a multidisciplinary approach as not clinically relevant and compatible with a participation in the clinical study.
• Physical examination without any clinical findings of clinical relevance (per medical/anesthesia staffs judgment) that could compromise participation in the clinical study or could affect the collection and/or evaluation of the study parameters. The findings of clinical relevance considered as contraindications to SPVN06 treatment include, but are not limited to, pulmonary pathology such as COPD, asthma, cardiac conditions such as congestive heart failure or valve disease, renal issues such as renal insufficiency and endocrine issues such as diabetes.

Exclusion Criteria
Subjects are not eligible to participate in this study if any of the following criteria apply:

• Subjects with prior administration of any gene therapy or any previous treatment with stem cell therapy for ocular or nonocular disease.
• Subjects participating in another clinical trial and receiving an investigational medicinal product (IMP) within five half-lives or 90 days prior to the injection of SPVN06.
• Subjects with RCD due to any mutation in genes other than those listed in the inclusion criteria.

- Subjects with systemic disease or other pathology not related to their diagnosis of RCD, and whose symptoms or associated treatments may affect vision, for example cancers or pathology of the central nervous system.
- Subjects with narrow iridocorneal angles or any other medical situation contraindicating pupillary dilation.
- Subjects known to be allergic to any of the delivery vehicle constituents or to any other drugs planned to be used during the clinical study.
- Subjects with known allergies to corticosteroids, or who will be unable to tolerate the corticosteroid regimen as described in the protocol.
- Subjects with systemic disease or other medical or psychiatric conditions that preclude safe participation in the study.
- Subjects receiving immunosuppressive therapies, other than the immune modulating regimen described in this protocol, or any other therapy known to influence the immune system including but not limited to steroid implants, cytostatics, interferons, tumor necrosis factor (TNF)-binding proteins, drugs acting on immunophilins, or antibodies with known impact on the immune system.
- Subjects of reproductive potential unwilling to use effective contraception starting right after ICF signature and for 12 months after SPVN06 SRI.
- Subjects who are pregnant or breastfeeding.
- Subjects who are unwilling or unable (based on the investigator's judgment) to comply with the study protocol.
- Subjects with any condition that would not allow them to complete follow-up examinations during the study and, in the opinion of the investigator, would make them unsuitable for the study.
- Subjects positive for human immunodeficiency virus (HIV) or any other systemic immunocompromising disease.
- Subjects who have undergone, within 6 months before inclusion, any significant ocular surgery (per investigator's judgment) that could interfere with the evaluation of SPVN06 study objectives.
- Presence of eye disorders that could interfere with the assessment of visual acuity and/or any other ocular assessments, including SD-OCT, during the study.
- Presence of any systemic or ocular diseases, other than nonsyndromic retinitis pigmentosa (RP), that can cause vision loss.
- Prior vitrectomy or vitreomacular surgery.
- Presence of vitreomacular adhesion or traction, epiretinal membrane macular pucker or macular hole, evident by ophthalmoscopy and/or SD-OCT examinations and assessed by the investigator to significantly affect central vision.
- Current evidence of retinal detachment assessed by the investigator to significantly affect central vision.
- Active ocular inflammation or recurrent history of idiopathic or autoimmune-associated uveitis.
- Subjects with presence of any suspected or active ocular or periocular infection (conjunctivitis, keratitis, scleritis, and endophthalmitis).
- Subjects with history of glaucoma.

- Subjects with uncontrolled intraocular pressure (IOP).
- Subjects with active cancer or currently receiving any therapy for cancer treatment.
- Subjects with any history of ocular malignancy.
- Subjects with a clinically significant cardiac disease on routine clinical examination (history, physical examination), or known congestive heart failure, myocardial infarction, clinically significant valvular heart disease, clinically significant cardiac rhythm or conduction abnormalities.
- Subjects with unstable/uncontrolled hypertension, defined by national recommendations.
- Subjects with pulmonary dysfunction or severe obstructive pulmonary disease.
- Subjects with active tuberculosis.
- Subjects with liver or renal insufficiency.
- Subjects with unstable endocrine disease, including unstable diabetes or thyroid disease.
- Subjects with active Hepatitis B or Hepatitis C.
- Subjects with clinically active infection of herpetic diseases, including herpes simplex virus, varicella zoster virus (VZV), cytomegalovirus (CMV) or EBV.
- Subjects with known history of ocular infection with herpes simplex virus.
- Subjects with active (extraocular) infection (requiring or not the prolonged or chronic use of antimicrobial agents).
- Immunocompromised subjects with previous solid organ or bone marrow transplant.
- Subjects who receive a live vaccine less than 4 weeks prior to SPVN06 injection.
- Subjects who were infected by COVID-19 less than 2 weeks prior to SPVN06 injection.
- Subjects who have recently received (less than 4 weeks) or plan to receive a COVID-19 vaccination.
- Incapacitated subjects, as defined by national laws.

Ages Eligible for Study
18 years and older (Adult, Older Adult)

Sexes Eligible for Study
All

Accepts Healthy Volunteers
No

Primary purpose: Treatment
Allocation: Randomized
Interventional model: Parallel assignment
Interventional model description: Phase I/II study including an open-label dose-escalation phase (Step 1) and a three-arm, controlled, double-masked, randomized extension phase (Step 2)
Masking: Quadruple (Participant Care Provider Investigator Outcomes Assessor)

Masking Description: Phase I/II study including an open-label dose-escalation phase (Step 1) and a three-arm, controlled, double-masked, randomized extension phase (Step 2). In Cohorts 5 and 6 of Step 2, subjects and the designated study personnel will be masked to subject's dose assignment. Cohort 4 (untreated group) will be unmasked.

Arms and Interventions

Participant group/arm	Intervention/treatment
Experimental: Step 1: SPVN06 dose 1 participants will receive a single subretinal injection of SPVN06 dose 1 on day 0.	Drug: SPVN06 • AAV-RdCVF-RdCVFL
Experimental: Step 1: SPVN06 dose 2 Participants will receive a single subretinal injection of SPVN06 dose 2 on day 0	Drug: SPVN06 • AAV-RdCVF-RdCVFL
Experimental: Step 1: SPVN06 dose 3 Participants will receive a single subretinal injection of SPVN06 dose 3 on day 0	Drug: SPVN06 • AAV-RdCVF-RdCVFL
Experimental: Step 2: SPVN06 dose recommended 1 Participants will receive a single subretinal injection of SPVN06 recommended dose 1 on day 0	Drug: SPVN06 • AAV-RdCVF-RdCVFL
Experimental: Step 2: SPVN06 dose recommended 2 Participants will receive a single subretinal injection of SPVN06 recommended dose 2 on day 0	Drug: SPVN06 • AAV-RdCVF-RdCVFL
No intervention: Step 2: Control group	

Primary outcome measures

Outcome measure	Measure description	Time frame
Evaluation of the safety and tolerability of a single injection of SPVN06 in subjects with advanced RCD due to a mutation in the RHO, PDE6A, or PDE6B gene, 12 months after administration of gene therapy	Incidence and severity of systemic and ocular AEs and SAEs	Baseline to 12 months after administration of gene therapy

Secondary outcome measures

Outcome measure	Measure description	Time frame
Evaluation of the long-term safety and tolerability of a single injection of SPVN06 in subjects with advanced RCD due to a mutation in the RHO, PDE6A, or PDE6B gene, up to 5 years after treatment administration	Incidence and severity of systemic and ocular AEs and SAEs	Up to 5 years after treatment
Evaluation of viral shedding and biodissemination up to 6 months after treatment administration	Quantification of viral DNA copies in tears (viral shedding) and in blood (biodissemination)	Up to 6 months after treatment
Evaluation of the immune response against the viral vector of SPVN06 up to 5 years after treatment administration	Titration of total antibodies against the viral capsid	Up to 5 years after treatment
Evaluation of preliminary efficacy as assessed by visual acuity	BCVA change from baseline (EDTRS chart)	Up to 5 years after treatment

Evaluation of preliminary efficacy as assessed by optical coherence tomography	Anatomical change from baseline (SD-OCT)	Up to 5 years after treatment
Evaluation of preliminary efficacy as assessed by color vision	Change from baseline of parameters collected by Cambridge and Lanthony tests	Up to 5 years after treatment
Evaluation of preliminary efficacy as assessed by visual field	Change from baseline of static perimetry, kinetic perimetry, and microperimetry	Up to 5 years after treatment
Evaluation of preliminary efficacy as assessed by retinal sensitivity	Change from baseline of parameters collected by full-field electroretinography	Up to 5 years after treatment
Evaluation of preliminary efficacy as assessed by retinal sensitivity	Change from baseline of parameters collected by FST	Up to 5 years after treatment
Evaluation of preliminary efficacy as assessed by FAF	Change from baseline of parameters collected by fundus autofluorescence	Up to 5 years after treatment
Evaluation of preliminary efficacy as assessed by adaptive optics imaging	Change from baseline of parameters collected by RTX1 and AOSLO	Up to 5 years after treatment
Evaluation of preliminary efficacy as assessed by quality of life	Change from baseline of parameters collected by VFQ-25	Up to 5 years after treatment
Evaluation of preliminary efficacy as assessed by quality of life	Change from baseline of parameters collected by ViSIO-PRO	Up to 5 years after treatment

Other outcome measures

Outcome measure	Measure description	Time frame
Exploratory objective	Collect and store urine and blood (in addition to the body fluids used for the assessment of viral shedding and biodissemination) for further exploration of biomarkers of medical interest not already identified at time of protocol submission	Up to 5 years after treatment

Sponsor
SparingVision

Collaborators
No information provided

Investigators
No information provided

General Publications
No publications available

Recruiting

United States/Europe

Dose-Escalation Study to Evaluate the Safety and Tolerability of GS030 in Subjects with Retinitis Pigmentosa (PIONEER)

ClinicalTrials.gov ID NCT03326336

Sponsor GenSight Biologics
Information provided by GenSight Biologics (Responsible Party)
Last Update Posted 2022-07-26

Brief Summary
The objective of this study is to evaluate the safety and tolerability of escalating doses of a gene therapy called GS030-DP (injected study treatment) administered via a single intravitreal injection and repeated light stimulation using a medical device called GS030-MD (stimulating glasses) in subjects with documented diagnosis of nonsyndromic Retinitis Pigmentosa.

Official Title
A Phase 1/2a, Open-Label, Nonrandomized, Dose-Escalation Study to Evaluate the Safety and Tolerability of GS030 in Subjects With Retinitis Pigmentosa.

Conditions
Nonsyndromic Retinitis Pigmentosa

Intervention/Treatment
Combination Product: Gene therapy: GS030-DP and Medical device: GS030-MD

Study Start (Actual)
2018-09-26

Primary Completion (Estimated)
2022-12

Study Completion (Estimated)
2025-12

Enrollment (Estimated)
15

Study Type
Interventional

Phase
Phase 1 Phase 2

Other Study ID Numbers
GS030_CLIN_001
2017-002204-27 (EudraCT Number)

Study Contact
Name: Magali Taiel, MD
Phone Number: +33 (0)7 62 89 12 52
Email: mtaiel@gensight-biologics.com

Study Contact Backup
Name: Michel Roux, MD
Phone Number: +33 (0)1 76 21 72 36
Email: mroux@gensight-biologics.com
United States
Pennsylvania Locations

Pittsburgh, Pennsylvania, United States, 15213
Recruiting
UPMC Eye Center

Contact
Joseph Martel, MD
412-647-3434
Principal Investigator:
Joseph Martel, MD

France

Paris, France, 75012
Recruiting
Centre Hospitalier National d'Ophtalmologie (CHNP) des Quinze-Vingts

Contact
Elise BOULANGER-SCEMAMA, MD
+33665895460 eboulanger@for.paris
Principal Investigator:
Elise BOULANGER-SCEMAMA, MD

United Kingdom

London, United Kingdom
Recruiting
Moorfields Eye Hospital NHS Foundation Trust, 162 City Road

Contact
Simona ESPOSTI, Dr.

Contact
s.esposti@nhs.net
Principal Investigator:
Simona ESPOSTI, MD

Eligibility Criteria
Main selection criteria:

- Age ≥ 18 years to ≤75 years at the time of ICF signature.

- Diagnosis of nonsyndromic RP is defined as:
  - Clinical diagnosis of nonsyndromic RP based on history, midperipheral visual dysfunction, and fundoscopic appearance.
  - Diagnosis of nonsyndromic RP is confirmed on full-field ERG
- Visual acuity:
  - Visual acuity in the dose-escalation cohorts of no better LP.
  - Visual acuity in the extension cohort of no better than CF pending review of dose-escalation cohort data by the DSMB.
- Relatively preserved ganglion cell layer volume and retinal nerve fiber layer thickness, as measured with spectral domain optical coherence tomography (SD-OCT).
- Interpupillary distance of ≥51 mm and ≤ 72 mm.
- Refractive error of the study eye between −6 diopters and + 6 diopters.

Main nonselection criteria:

- Prior receipt of any gene therapy.
- Subjects who have undergone significant ocular surgery (per investigator determination) within 3 months prior to Visit 1.
- Presence of narrow iridocorneal angles contraindicating pupillary dilation.
- Presence of disorders of the ocular media which interfere with visual acuity and other ocular assessments, including SD-OCT, during the study period.
- Presence of any systemic or ocular diseases, or pathologies, other than non-syndromic RP, or their associated therapies, that can cause or have the potential to cause vision loss.
- Prior vitrectomy or vitreomacular surgery.
- Presence of vitreomacular adhesion or traction, epiretinal membrane, macular pucker and macular hole, evident by ophthalmoscopy and/or by SD-OCT examinations and assessed by the investigator to significantly affect central vision.
- Current evidence of retinal detachment assessed by the investigator to significantly affect central vision.
- Active ocular inflammation or recurrent history of idiopathic or autoimmune associated uveitis.
- Presence of an Active Implantable Medical Device.
- Subjects who have undergone thermal laser procedure to the retina within 3 months of trial entry, or any prior thermal laser procedure to the macular region.

Ages Eligible for Study
18–75 years (Adult, Older Adult)

Sexes Eligible for Study
All

Accepts Healthy Volunteers
No

Design Details
Primary Purpose: Treatment
Allocation: N/A
Interventional Model: Sequential Assignment
Interventional Model Description: 3 dose-escalation cohorts with 3 subjects per each cohort plus 1 extension cohort at the highest well-tolerated dose.
Masking: None (Open Label)

Arms and interventions

Participant group/arm	Intervention/treatment
Other: Cohort 3 dose escalation cohorts (low, medium and high dose) with three subjects per cohort followed by an extension cohort at the highest well-tolerated dose with 3–9 subjects	Combination product: Gene therapy: GS030-DP and medical device: GS030-MD • GS030-drug product (GS030-DP)—recombinant adeno-associated viral vector, derived from serotype 2 (rAAV2.7 m8), containing the optimized channel rhodopsin ChrimsonR-tdTomato gene under the control of the ubiquitous CAG promoter (rAAV2.7 m8-CAG-ChrimsonR-tdTomato) GS030-medical device (GS030-MD)—visual interface stimulating glasses (that amplify the external visual stimulus to the optogenetically engineered retina)

Primary outcome measures

Outcome measure	Measure description	Time frame
The safety and tolerability of escalating doses of GS030-DP administered via a single IVT and repeated light stimulation using GS030-MD in subjects with nonsyndromic retinitis Pigmentosa	Safety and tolerability of GS030 treatment at week 52/year 1, by assessments based on local and systemic safety issues, specifically those related to IVT of GS030-DP and the subsequent repeated use of GS030-MD, as assessed by incidence of adverse events	Week 52/ year 1

Secondary outcome measures

Outcome measure	Measure description	Time frame
Evaluate the treatment effect of GS030 as assessed by visual acuity	Assessment of the treatment effect with the change from baseline to week 52 of parameters measured with the Freiburg Visual Acuity & Contrast Test (FrACT) free computer program that uses graphics capabilities and psychometric methods to provide automated, self-paced measurement and the full field threshold stimulus test (FST) measuring the illuminance necessary to stimulate the most sensitive parts of the retina, and thus determines a quantifiable stimulation threshold (before and after gene transfer, with GS030-MD turned ON and turned OFF)	Week 52/ year 1

Evaluate the treatment effect of GS030 as assessed by visual function	Assessment of the treatment effect with the change from baseline to week 52 of parameters measured with Humphrey visual field 10–2 standardized automated perimetry, square localization test, displaying white square at a random location on a black background and direction of motion test measuring the ability of subjects to determine the direction of an object moving in the visual field (before and after gene transfer, with GS030-MD turned ON and turned OFF)	Week 52/ year 1
Evaluate the treatment effect of GS030 as assessed by mobility	Assessment of the treatment effect with the change from baseline to week 52 of parameters measured with door task (before and after gene transfer, with GS030-MD turned ON and turned OFF)	Week 52/ year 1
Evaluate the treatment effect of GS030 as assessed by mobility	Assessment of the treatment effect with the change from baseline to week 52 of parameters measured with line task (before and after gene transfer, with GS030-MD turned ON and turned OFF)	Week 52/ year 1
Evaluate the treatment effect of GS030 as assessed by QoL	Assessment of the treatment effect on quality of life changes from baseline to week 52 with the visual functioning Questionnaire-25 (VFQ-25). VFQ25 is a 25-item questionnaire with 47 questions, each question has several responses scored on a scale from 0 to 5, 0 to 6, or 0 to 10. Values are calculated in percentages	Week 52/ year 1
Evaluate the treatment effect of GS030 as assessed by QoL	Assessment of the treatment effect on quality of life changes from baseline to week 52 with the short form survey 36 version 2 (SF-36v2). The SF-36v2 is a subject-rated 36-item questionnaire assessing subject health. There are eight scaled scores, which are the weighted sums of the questions in their section. Each scale is directly transformed into a 0–100 scale. A lower score indicates more disability, and a higher score indicates less disability (a score of 0 is equivalent to maximum disability, and a score of 100 is equivalent to no disability)	Week 52/ year 1
Evaluate immune response to recombinant adeno associated viral vector, derived from serotype 2 (rAAV2.7 m8) and ChR tdT protein	Immune response to rAAV2.7 m8 and ChR-tdT protein from baseline to week 52	Week 52/ year 1

Sponsor
GenSight Biologics

Collaborators
No information provided

Investigators
No information provided

General Publications
No publications available

Recruiting

United States/Canada/Europe/Israel

Gene Therapy Trial for the Treatment of X-Linked Retinitis Pigmentosa Associated with Variants in the RPGR Gene

ClinicalTrials.gov ID NCT04671433

Sponsor MeiraGTx UK II Ltd.
Information provided by MeiraGTx UK II Ltd. (Responsible Party)
Last Update Posted 2023-09-13

Brief Summary
A clinical trial of AAV5-RPGR vector for patients with X-linked retinitis pigmentosa (XLRP).

Official Title
Phase 3 Randomized, Controlled Study of AAV5-RPGR for the Treatment of X-linked Retinitis Pigmentosa Associated With Variants in the RPGR Gene

Conditions
X-linked retinitis pigmentosa

Intervention/treatment
Biological: Genetic: AAV5-RPGR
Biological: Genetic: AAV5-RPGR

Study Start (Actual)
2021-03-16

Primary Completion (Estimated)
2024-03

Study Completion (Estimated)
2024-03

Enrollment (Estimated)
96

Study Type
Interventional

Phase
Phase 3

Other Study ID Numbers
MGT-RPGR-021

Name: MeiraGTx Clinical Project Manager
Phone Number: +44 (0)203866 4320
Email: info@lumeosstudy.com
United States
California Locations

Los Angeles, California, United States, 90027
Recruiting
Children's Hospital Los Angeles

Contact
Aaron L Nagiel, MD, PhD
323-361-7194 anagiel@chla.usc.edu

Contact
Hiliary Schwartz
+13233611004 hschwartz@chla.usc.edu

Palo Alto, California, United States, 94303
Recruiting
Stanford University

Contact
Vinit Mahajan, MD, PhD
650-497-1182 vinit.mahajan@stanford.edu

Contact
Mark Santos
650497-7935 mark.santos@stanford.edu

San Diego, California, United States, 92093-0946
Recruiting
Shiley Eye Institute, University of California San Diego

Contact
Shyamanga Borooah, MD
858-822-2585 sborooah@health.ucsd.edu

Contact
Ilaina Molina
8588222585 imolina@health.ucsd.edu

Florida Locations

Gainesville, Florida, United States, 32607
Recruiting
Vitreo Retinal Associates

Contact
Christine Kay, MD
352-371-2800 christine@vra-pa.com

Contact
Jing Zang, MD
352-665-6672 JingZhang@vra-pa.com

Georgia Locations

Atlanta, Georgia, United States, 30322
Recruiting
The Emory Eye Centre

Contact
Nieraj Jain, MD
404-778-5816 nieraj.jain@emory.edu

Contact
Judith Tribe
jtribe@emory.edu

Massachusetts Locations

Boston, Massachusetts, United States, 02114
Recruiting
Massachusetts Eye and Ear, Centre for Clinical Research Operations

Contact
Rachel Huckfeldt, MD
617-573-6060 Rachel_Huckfeldt@meei.Harvard.Edu

Contact
Mirjana Nordmann, PhD
617-573-6060 Mirjana_Nordmann@MEEI.HARVARD.EDU

Michigan Locations

Ann Arbor, Michigan, United States, 48105
Recruiting
University of Michigan, W.K. Kellogg Eye Centre

Contact
Thomas Wubben, MD
734-763-8122 twubben@med.umich.edu

Contact
Sheila Gilbert
734-936-9798 slreeves@med.umich.edu

North Carolina Locations

Durham, North Carolina, United States, 22710
Recruiting
Duke Eye Center

Contact
Lejla Vajzovic, MD
919-668-5316 lejla.vajzovic@duke.edu

Contact
Carol White
919613-5078 carol.white302@duke.edu

Pennsylvania Locations

Pittsburgh, Pennsylvania, United States, 15213
Recruiting
University of Pittsburgh Medical Centre

Contact
Kunal Dansingani, MD
412-647-8030 dansinganik@upmc.edu

Contact
Dipanwita Samanta
+14126473928 samantad@upmc.edu

Texas Locations

Bellaire, Texas, United States, 77401
Recruiting
Retinal Consultants of Houston

Contact
David Brown, MD
713-524-3434 dmbmd@houstonretina.com

Contact
Chelsey Moore
713-394-7575 chelsey.moore@houstonretina.com

Belgium

Ghent, Belgium, 9000
Recruiting
Ghent University Hospital

Contact
Bart Peter Leroy, MD, PhD
+32 93326344 bart.leroy@uzgent.be

Contact
Julie Sambaer
+32 9332 16 74 Julie.Sambaer@uzgent.be

Canada
Ontario Locations

Toronto, Ontario, Canada, M5G 1X8
Recruiting
The Hospital for Sick Children

Contact
Elise Heon, MD
416-813-7654 elise.heon@sickkids.ca

Contact
Sabahat Javaid
416-813-7654 ext. 301511 sabahat.javaid@sickkids.ca

Denmark

Glostrup, Denmark, 2600
Recruiting
Rigshospitalet Glostrup

Contact
Line Kessel, Prof.
+454160 2712 line.kessel.01@regionh.dk

Contact
Ulla Birch Flensborg
+453863 4814 ulla.birch.flensborg@regionh.dk

France

Paris, France, 75012
Recruiting
Centre Hospitalier National d'Ophtalmologie (CHNO) des Quinze-Vingts

Contact
Isabelle Audo, Prof.
+33140 02 14 55 isabelle.audo@inserm.fr

Contact
Thilissa Dib
+33 1 40 02 14 55 tdib@15-20.fr

Israel

Jerusalem, Israel, 91120
Recruiting
Hadassah Medical Center

Contact
Eyal Banin, MD
+9722677 6585 banine@mail.huji.ac.il

Contact
Einav Nahmany
+972 508538865 einavnahmany@gmail.com

Italy

Florence, Italy
Recruiting
Azienda Ospedaliero, Universitaria Careggi

Contact
Fabrizio Giansanti, Prof
fabrizio.giansanti@unifi.it

Contact
Ilaria Biagini
ilaria.biagini55@gmail.com

Milan, Italy
Recruiting
Ospedale San Paolo di Milano

Contact
Luca Mario Rossetti, Dr.
luca.rossetti@ao-sanpaolo.it

Contact
Leonardo Colombo, Dr.
leonardo.colombo.82@gmail.com

Napoli, Italy
Recruiting
AOU Università degli, Studi della Campania

Contact
Francesca Simonelli, Prof
Francesca.Simonelli@unicampania.it

Contact
Carmela Acerra
carmela.acerra@unicampania.it

Roma, Italy
Recruiting
IRCCS Fondazione G. B. Bietti, Ospedale Britannico

Contact
Lucia Ziccardi, Dr.
lucia.ziccardi@fondazionebietti.it

Contact
Federica Petrocchi
federica.petrocchi@fondazionebietti.it

Netherlands

Amsterdam, Netherlands, 1105AZ
Recruiting
Amsterdam UMC

Contact
Camiel Boon, MD
+31 20 56 68618 camiel.boon@amsterdamumc.nl

Contact
Monique Wezel
+31 20 56 68618 m.wezel@amsterdamumc.nl

Nijmegen, Netherlands, 6525EX
Recruiting
Radboud University Medical Center

Contact
Carel Hoyng, MD
+31 243613138 Carel.Hoyng@radboudumc.nl

Contact
Alexandra Versleijen
+31 243613212 Alexandra.versleijen@radboudumc.nl

Spain

Madrid, Spain, 28040
Recruiting
University Hospital Fundación Jiménez Díaz

Contact
Blanca Garcia-Sandoval, Dr.
+34915504800 ext. 2110 bgarcia@fjd.es

Contact
Ana Lorena Perez Hernandez
+34915504876 ext. 2110 ALPerezH@quironsalud.es

Switzerland

Basel, Switzerland, 4031
Recruiting
University Hospital Basel

Contact
Hendrik Scholl, Prof.
+41612658651 Hendrik.Scholl@usb.ch

Contact
Daniela Hauenstein
+41612658718 Daniela.Hauenstein@usb.ch

Lausanne, Switzerland, 1004
Recruiting
Hôpital Ophtalmique Jules-Gonin

Contact
Hoai Viet Tran, Dr.
+41 21626 88 50 hoaiviet.tran@fa2.ch

Contact
Aurelie Navarro
+41 21626 81 66 aurelie.navarro@fa2.ch

United Kingdom

Edinburgh, United Kingdom, EH3 9HA
Recruiting
NHS Lothian

Contact
Roly Megaw, Dr.
+447890 566708 roly.megaw@nhslothian.scot.nhs.uk

Contact
Margaret L Mcdonald
+447890 566708 margaret.l.mcdonald@nhslothian.scot.nhs.uk

Glasgow, United Kingdom, G12 0YN
Recruiting
Glasgow Centre for Ophthalmic Research, Gartnaval General Hospital

Contact
David Gilmour, Prof.
+441412112523 David.Gilmour@ggc.scot.nhs.uk

Contact
Clodagh Duffy
+441412111037 Clodagh.Duffy@ggc.scot.nhs.uk

Leeds, United Kingdom, LS9 7TF
Recruiting
Leeds Centre for Ophthalmology, St James' University Hospital

Contact
Raj Mukherjee, Dr.
+44 (0)1132065084 raj.mukherjee@nhs.net

Contact
Rabiya Ali
+44 (0)1132065084 rabiya.ali@nhs.net

London, United Kingdom, EC1V 2PD
Recruiting
Moorfield Eye Hospital (MEH)

Contact
James Bainbridge, MD
+44 207253 3411 james.bainbridge1@nhs.net

Contact
Sarah Hill
+44(0) 2075663411 Ext 2873 sarah.hill79@nhs.net

Eligibility Criteria
Inclusion Criteria
- Male or female
- 3 years of age or older
- Has XLRP confirmed by a retinal specialist and has a predicted disease-causing sequence variant in RPGR confirmed by an accredited laboratory.

Exclusion Criteria
Show less

Ages Eligible for Study
3 years and older (Child, Adult, Older Adult)

Sexes Eligible for Study
All

Accepts Healthy Volunteers
No

Design Details
Primary purpose: Treatment
Allocation: Randomized
Interventional model: Parallel assignment
Interventional model description: Bilateral, subretinal administration of AAV5-RPGR—immediate treatment group
Masking: Single (Outcomes Assessor)
Masking description: No intervention—deferred treatment group (Bilateral, subretinal administration of AAV5-RPGR to be administered in the follow-up study)

Arms and interventions

Participant group/arm	Intervention/treatment
Experimental: Experimental—immediate treatment RPGR4e11	Biological: Genetic: AAV5-RPGR • Bilateral, subretinal administration of AAV5-RPGR—immediate treatment group Biological: Genetic: AAV5-RPGR • No intervention—deferred treatment group (bilateral, sub-retinal administration of AAV5-RPGR to be administered in the follow-up study)
Other: Deferred treatment Deferred treatment	Biological: Genetic: AAV5-RPGR • Bilateral, sub-retinal administration of AAV5-RPGR—immediate treatment group Biological: Genetic: AAV5-RPGR • No intervention—deferred treatment group (bilateral, sub-retinal administration of AAV5-RPGR to be administered in the follow-up study)
Active comparator: Experimental immediate treatment RPGR2e11	Biological: Genetic: AAV5-RPGR • Bilateral, sub-retinal administration of AAV5-RPGR—immediate treatment group Biological: Genetic: AAV5-RPGR • No intervention—deferred treatment group (bilateral, sub-retinal administration of AAV5-RPGR to be administered in the follow-up study)

Primary outcome measures

Outcome measure	Measure description	Time frame
Change from baseline to week 52 in vision-guided mobility assessment (VMA) as measured by the ability of the participant to navigate through a VMA maze	Change from baseline to week 52 in vision-guided mobility assessment (VMA) as measured by the ability of the participant to navigate through a VMA maze	52 weeks

Secondary outcome measures

Outcome measure	Measure description	Time frame
Change in retinal function as assessed by mean retinal sensitivity within the central 10 degrees (MRS10) in static perimetry at week 52	Mean retinal sensitivity within the central 10 degrees (MRS10) in static perimetry at week 52	Day 1—week 52
Change in retinal function as assessed by pointwise responder in full visual field at week 52	Pointwise responder in full visual field at week 52	Day 1—week 52
Change in retinal function as assessed by pointwise responder in the central 30 degrees visual field at week 52	Pointwise responder in the central 30 degrees visual field at week 52	Day 1—week 52
Change in retinal function as assessed by mean retinal sensitivity within the full visual field (MRS90) in static perimetry at week 52	Mean retinal sensitivity within the full visual field (MRS90) in static perimetry at week 52	Day 1—week 52
Change in functional vision as measured by patient-reported outcomes at week 52	Change in functional vision as measured by patient-reported outcomes at week 52	Day 1—week 52

Change in visual function as assessed by binocular low luminance visual acuity using the early treatment diabetic retinopathy study (ETDRS) chart letter score at week 52	Binocular low luminance visual acuity using the ETDRS chart letter score at week 52	Day 1—week 52
Change in visual function as assessed by binocular best corrected visual acuity (BCVA) using the early treatment diabetic retinopathy study (ETDRS) chart letter score at week 52	Binocular BCVA using the ETDRS chart letter score at week 52	Day 1—week 52
Safety and tolerability through week 52 as assessed by:	• Number of participants with ocular and nonocular adverse events • Number of participants with abnormalities in hematologic and clinical chemistry parameters	Day 1—week 52

Collaborators and investigators

Sponsor
MeiraGTx UK II Ltd.

Collaborators
- Janssen Research & Development, LLC

Investigators
- Principal Investigator: James Bainbridge, MD, Moorfield Eye Hospital (MEH)

General Publications
No publications available

Recruiting

United States/Canada/Europe/Israel

Follow-Up Gene Therapy Trial for the Treatment of X-Linked Retinitis Pigmentosa Associated with Variants in the RPGR Gene

ClinicalTrials.gov ID NCT04794101

Sponsor MeiraGTx UK II Ltd.
Information provided by MeiraGTx UK II Ltd. (Responsible Party)
Last Update Posted 2023-09-13

Brief Summary
A clinical trial of AAV5-RPGR vector for patients with X-linked retinitis pigmentosa (XLRP).

Official Title
Follow-up Phase 3 Randomized, Controlled Study of AAV5-RPGR for the Treatment of X-linked Retinitis Pigmentosa Associated with Variants in the RPGR Gene

Conditions
X-Linked retinitis pigmentosa
Intervention/treatment
Biological: Genetic: AAV5-RPGR 4e11
Biological: Genetic: AAV5-RPGR 2e11

Study Start (Actual)
2021-03-16

Primary Completion (Estimated)
2029-05

Study Completion (Estimated)
2029-05

Enrollment (Estimated)
96

Study Type
Interventional
Phase
Phase 3

Other Study ID Numbers
MGT-RPGR-022

Study Contact
Name: MeiraGTx Clinical Project Manager
Phone Number: +44 (0)203866 4320
Email: info@lumeosstudy.com
United States
California Locations

Los Angeles, California, United States, 90027
Recruiting
Children's Hospital Los Angeles

Contact
Aaron L Nagiel, MD, PhD
323-361-7194 anagiel@chla.usc.edu

Contact
Hiliary Schwartz
323-361-1004 hschwartz@chla.usc.edu

Palo Alto, California, United States, 94303
Recruiting
Stanford University

Contact
Vinit Mahajan, MD, PhD
650-497-1182 vinit.mahajan@stanford.edu

Contact
Mark Santos
650497-7935 mark.santos@stanford.edu

San Diego, California, United States, 92093-0946
Recruiting
Shiley Eye Institute, University of California San Diego

Contact
Shyamanga Borooah, MD
858-822-2585 sborooah@health.ucsd.edu

Contact
Iliana Milina
8588222585 imolina@health.ucsd.edu

Florida Locations

Gainesville, Florida, United States, 32607
Recruiting
Vitreo Retinal Associates

Contact
Christine Kay, MD
352-371-2800 christine@vra-pa.com

Contact
Jing Zang, MD
3526656672 JingZhang@vra-pa.com

Georgia Locations

Atlanta, Georgia, United States, 30322
Recruiting
The Emory Eye Centre

Contact
Nieraj E Jain, MD
404-778-5816 nieraj.jain@emory.edu

Contact
Judith Tribe
jtribe@emory.edu

Massachusetts Locations

Boston, Massachusetts, United States, 02114
Recruiting
Boston Eye and Ear

Contact
Rachel Huckfeldt, MD
617-573-6060 Rachel_Huckfeldt@meei.Harvard.Edu

Contact
Mirjana Nordmann, PhD
617-573-6060 Mirjana_Nordmann@MEEI.HARVARD.EDU

Michigan Locations

Ann Arbor, Michigan, United States, 48105
Recruiting
University of Michigan, W.K. Kellogg Eye Centre

Contact
Thomas Wubben, MD
734-763-8122 twubben@med.umich.edu

Contact
Sheila Gilbert
734-936-9798 slreeves@med.umich.edu

North Carolina Locations

Durham, North Carolina, United States, 22710
Recruiting
Duke Eye Center

Contact
Lejla Vajzovic, MD
919-668-5316 lejla.vajzovic@duke.edu

Contact
Carol White
919613-5078 carol.white302@duke.edu

Pennsylvania Locations

Pittsburgh, Pennsylvania, United States, 15213
Recruiting
University of Pittsburgh Medical Centre

Contact
Kunal Dansingani, MD
412-647-8030 dansinganik@upmc.edu

Contact
Dipanwita Samanta
4126473928 samantad@upmc.edu

Texas Locations

Bellaire, Texas, United States, 77401
Recruiting
Retinal Consultants of Houston

Contact
David Brown, MD
713-524-3434 dmbmd@houstonretina.com

Contact
Chelsey Moore
713-394-7575 chelsey.moore@houstonretina.com

Belgium

Ghent, Belgium, 9000
Recruiting
Ghent University Hospital

Contact
Bart Peter Leroy, MD, PhD
+32 93326344 bart.leroy@uzgent.be

Contact
Julie Sambaer
+32 9332 16 74 Julie.Sambaer@uzgent.be

Canada
Ontario Locations

Toronto, Ontario, Canada, M5G 1X8
Recruiting
The Hospital for Sick Children

Contact
Elise Heon, MD
416-813-7654 elise.heon@sickkids.ca

Contact
Sabahat Javaid
416-813-7654 ext. 301511 sabahat.javaid@sickkids.ca

Denmark

Glostrup, Denmark, 2600
Recruiting
Rigshospitalet Glostrup

Contact
Line Kessel, Prof.
+454160 2712 line.kessel.01@regionh.dk

Contact
Ulla Birch Flensborg
+453863 4814 ulla.birch.flensborg@regionh.dk

France

Paris, France, 75012
Recruiting
Centre Hospitalier National d'Ophtalmologie (CHNO) des Quinze-Vingts

Contact
Isabelle Audo, Prof.
+33140 02 14 55 isabelle.audo@inserm.fr

Contact
Thilissa Dib
+33 1 40 02 14 55 tdib@15-20.fr

Israel

Jerusalem, Israel, 91120
Recruiting
Hadassah Medical Center

Contact
Eyal Banin, MD
+9722677 6585 banine@mail.huji.ac.il

Contact
Einav Nahmany
+972 508538,865 einavnahmany@gmail.com

Italy

Florence, Italy
Recruiting
Azienda Ospedaliero, Universitaria Careggi

Contact
Fabrizio Giansanti, Prof
fabrizio.giansanti@unifi.it

Contact
Ilaria Biagini
ilaria.biagini55@gmail.com

Milan, Italy
Recruiting
Ospedale San Paolo di Milano

Contact
Luca Mario Rossetti, Dr.
luca.rossetti@ao-sanpaolo.it

Contact
Leonardo Colombo, Dr.
leonardo.colombo.82@gmail.com

Napoli, Italy
Recruiting
AOU Università degli, Studi della Campania

Contact
Francesca Simonelli, Prof
Francesca.Simonelli@unicampania.it

Contact
Carmela Acerra
carmela.acerra@unicampania.it

Roma, Italy
Recruiting
IRCCS Fondazione G. B. Bietti, Ospedale Britannico

Contact
Lucia Ziccardi, Dr.
lucia.ziccardi@fondazionebietti.it

Contact
Federica Petrocchi
federica.petrocchi@fondazionebietti.it

Netherlands
Amsterdam, Netherlands, 1105AZ
Recruiting
Amsterdam UMC

Contact
Camiel Boon, MD
+31 20 56 68618 camiel.boon@amsterdamumc.nl

Contact
Monique Wezel
+31 20 56 68618 m.wezel@amsterdamumc.nl

Nijmegen, Netherlands, 6525EX
Recruiting
Radboud University Medical Center

Contact
Carel Hoyng, MD
+31 243613138 Carel.Hoyng@radboudumc.nl

Contact
Alexandra Versleijen
+31 243613212 Alexandra.versleijen@radboudumc.nl

Spain

Madrid, Spain, 28040
Recruiting
University Hospital Fundación Jiménez Díaz

Contact
Blanca Garcia-Sandoval, Dr.
+34915504800 ext. 2110 bgarcia@fjd.es

Contact
Ana Lorena Perez Hernandez
+34915504876 ext. 2110 ALPerezH@quironsalud.es

Switzerland

Basel, Switzerland, 4031
Recruiting
University Hospital Basel

Contact
Hendrik Scholl, Prof.
+41612658651 Hendrik.Scholl@usb.ch

Contact
Daniela Hauenstein
+41612658718 Daniela.Hauenstein@usb.ch

Lausanne, Switzerland, 1004
Recruiting
Hôpital Ophtalmique Jules-Gonin

Contact
Hoai Viet Tran, Dr.
+41 21626 88 50 hoaiviet.tran@fa2.ch

Contact
Aurelie Navarro
+41 21626 81 66 aurelie.navarro@fa2.ch

United Kingdom

Edinburgh, United Kingdom, EH3 9HA
Recruiting
NHS Lothian

Contact
Roly Megaw, Dr.
+447890 566708 roly.megaw@nhslothian.scot.nhs.uk

Contact
Margaret L Mcdonald
+447890 566708 margaret.l.mcdonald@nhslothian.scot.nhs.uk

Glasgow, United Kingdom, G12 0YN
Recruiting
Glasgow Centre for Ophthalmic Research, Gartnaval General Hospital

Contact
David Gilmour, Prof.
+441412112523 David.Gilmour@ggc.scot.nhs.uk

Contact
Clodagh Duffy
+441412111037 Clodagh.Duffy@ggc.scot.nhs.uk

Leeds, United Kingdom, LS9 7TF
Recruiting
Leeds Centre for Ophthalmology, St James' University Hospital

Contact
Raj Mukherjee, Dr.
+44 (0)1132065084 raj.mukherjee@nhs.net

Contact
Rabiya Ali
+44 (0)1132065084 rabiya.ali@nhs.net

London, United Kingdom, EC1V 2PD
Recruiting
Moorfield Eye Hospital (MEH)

Contact
James Bainbridge, MD
+44 207253 3411 james.bainbridge@nhs.net

Contact
Sarah Hill
+44 (0) 2075663411 Ext.:2873 sarah.hill79@nhs.net

Eligibility Criteria
Inclusion Criteria

- Male or female 3 years of age or older has XLRP confirmed by a retinal specialist and has a predicted disease-causing sequence variant in RPGR confirmed by an accredited laboratory.

Exclusion Criteria
Ages Eligible for Study
3 Years and older (Child, Adult, Older Adult)

Sexes Eligible for Study
All

Accepts Healthy Volunteers
No

Design Details
Primary Purpose: Treatment
Allocation: Randomized
Interventional Model: Parallel Assignment
Interventional Model Description: 66 Patients randomized in MGT-RPGR-021.44 patients randomized to Immediate treatment arm. However, 22 patients randomized to the deferred arm. These patients will be treated in MGT-RPGR-022. All patients to be followed for 60 months.
Masking: Single (Outcomes Assessor)

Arms and interventions

Participant group/arm	Intervention/treatment
Experimental: Deferred treatment from MGT-RPGR-021 4e11 Deferred treatment	Biological: Genetic: AAV5-RPGR 4e11 • Bilateral, subretinal administration of AAV5-RPGR—deferred treatment group
Active comparator: Already treated in MGT-RPGR-021 Already treated	Biological: Genetic: AAV5-RPGR 4e11 • Bilateral, subretinal administration of AAV5-RPGR—deferred treatment group Biological: Genetic: AAV5-RPGR 2e11 • Bilateral, subretinal administration of AAV5-RPGR—deferred treatment group
Experimental: Deferred treatment from MGT-RPGR-021 2e11 Deferred treatment	Biological: Genetic: AAV5-RPGR 2e11 • Bilateral, subretinal administration of AAV5-RPGR—deferred treatment group

Primary outcome measures

Outcome measure	Measure description	Time frame
Change from baseline in vision-guided mobility assessment (VMA), as measured by the ability of the participant to navigate through a VMA maze, after bilateral subretinal delivery of AAV5-hRKp.RPGR	Change from baseline in vision-guided mobility assessment (VMA), as measured by the ability of the participant to navigate through a VMA maze, after bilateral subretinal delivery of AAV5-hRKp.RPGR	Day 1—month 60
Safety and tolerability of bilateral treatment through month 60 as assessed by:	• Number of participants with ocular and nonocular adverse events • Number of participants with abnormalities in hematologic and clinical chemistry parameters	Day 1—month 60

Secondary outcome measures

Outcome measure	Measure description	Time frame
Change in retinal function as assessed by mean retinal sensitivity within the central 10 degrees (MRS10)	Mean retinal sensitivity within the central 10 degrees (MRS10)	Day 1—month 60
Change in retinal function as assessed by pointwise responder in full visual field	Pointwise responder in full visual field	Day 1—month 60
Change in retinal function as assessed by pointwise responder in the central 30-degree visual field	Pointwise responder in the central 30-degree visual field	Day 1—month 60
Change in retinal function as assessed by mean retinal sensitivity within the full visual field (MRS90)	Mean retinal sensitivity within the full visual field (MRS90)	Day 1—month 60
Change in functional vision as measured by patient-reported outcomes	Change in functional vision as measured by patient-reported outcomes	Day 1—month 60
Change in visual function as assessed by binocular low luminance visual acuity using the early treatment diabetic retinopathy (ETDRS) chart letter score	Binocular low luminance visual acuity using the ETDRS chart letter score	Day 1—month 60
Change in visual function as assessed by binocular best corrected visual acuity (BCVA) using the early treatment diabetic retinopathy study (ETDRS) chart letter score	Binocular BCVA using the ETDRS chart letter score	Day 1—month 60

Sponsor
MeiraGTx UK II Ltd.

Collaborators
- Janssen Research & Development, LLC

Investigators
- Principal Investigator: James Bainbridge, MD, Moorfield Eye Hospital (MEH)

General Publications
No publications available

Recruiting

United States/United Kingdom

Long-Term Follow-Up Gene Therapy Study for XLRP RPGR

ClinicalTrials.gov ID NCT04312672

Sponsor MeiraGTx UK II Ltd.
Information provided by MeiraGTx UK II Ltd. (Responsible Party)
Last Update Posted 2022-12-06

Brief Summary
This a long-term follow-up study assessing safety of patients for up to 60 months following AAV2 vector in participants with XLRP caused by mutations in RPGR.

Official Title
Long-Term Follow-Up Study of Participants Following an Open Label, Multicentre, Phase I/II Dose Escalation Trial of a Recombinant Adeno-Associated Virus Vector (AAV2-RPGR) for Gene Therapy of Adults and Children With X-Linked Retinitis Pigmentosa Owing to Defects in Retinitis Pigmentosa GTPase Regulator (RPGR)

Conditions
X-linked retinitis pigmentosa

Intervention/Treatment
Biological: AAV-RPGR

Study Start (Actual)
2019-02-18

Primary Completion (Estimated)
2023-06

Study Completion (Estimated)
2023-06

Enrollment (Estimated)
36

Study Type
Observational

Other Study ID Numbers
MGT010

Study Contact
Name: Ocular Information
Phone number: +44203866 4320
Email: ocularinfo@meiragtx.com

United States
Massachusetts Locations

Boston, Massachusetts, United States, 02114
Recruiting
Massachusetts Eye and Ear Institute

Contact
Rachel Huckfeldt
rachel_huckfeldt@meei.harvard.edu

Michigan Locations

Ann Arbor, Michigan, United States, 48105
Recruiting
Kellogg Eye Center

Contact
Thomas Wubben
twubben@med.umich.edu

United Kingdom

Leeds, United Kingdom, LS9 7TF
Recruiting
Leeds Teaching Hospital

Contact
Martin McKibbin
martin.mckibbin@nhs.net

London, United Kingdom, EC1V 2PD
Recruiting
Moorfields Eye Hospital

Contact
James Bainbridge, MD
james.bainbridge1@nhs.net

Eligibility Criteria
Inclusion Criteria
- Received AAV2-RPGR in the MGT009 Study

Exclusion Criteria
- Unwilling or unable to meet with the requirements of the study

Study Population
Males receiving AAV2-RPGR in the MGT009 study

Ages Eligible for Study
5 Years and older (Child, Adult, Older Adult)

Sexes Eligible for Study
Male

Accepts Healthy Volunteers
No

Sampling Method
Nonprobability sample

Sponsor
MeiraGTx UK II Ltd.

Collaborators
No information provided

Investigators
No information provided

General Publications
No publications available

Recruiting

United States

Safety and Efficacy of rAAV2tYF-GRK1-RPGR in Subjects with X-Linked Retinitis Pigmentosa Caused by RPGR Mutations

ClinicalTrials.gov ID NCT03316560

Sponsor: Applied Genetic Technologies Corp
Information provided by Applied Genetic Technologies Corp (Responsible Party)
Last Update Posted 2021-07-15

Study Overview

Brief Summary
This study will evaluate the safety and efficacy of a recombinant adeno-associated virus vector (rAAV2tYF-GRK1-RPGR) in patients with X-linked retinitis pigmentosa caused by RPGR mutations.

Detailed Description
This study includes a nonrandomized, open-label, Phase 1/2 dose escalation portion, and a Phase 2 randomized, controlled, masked dose expansion portion.

Approximately 30 participants will be enrolled into the dose escalation portion of the study. Each participant will receive the study agent by subretinal injection in one eye on a single occasion. Enrollment will begin with the lowest dose and will proceed to higher doses only after review of safety data by a Data and Safety Monitoring Committee (DSMC). Within groups 1 through 3 and 5 and 6, enrollment of participants will be staggered by at least 2 weeks to allow adequate time for review of safety information by the investigators and sponsor. Within Group 4, enrollment of the first three pediatric participants will be staggered by at least 2 weeks to allow adequate time for review of safety information by the investigators and sponsor. Study agent administration will occur on Day 0. There are a total of 15 visits over approximately 36 months, and long-term follow-up evaluations annually at years 4 and 5.

After the phase 1/2 portion of the study is completed, approximately 12 participants, who were not part of the Phase 1/2 portion of the study, will be enrolled into the dose expansion portion of the study. These participants will be randomized in a 1:1 ratio to 1 of 2 treatment groups (i.e., Group 1 [low dose] and Group 2 [high dose]). Each participant will receive the assigned dose of AGTC-501 in one eye on a single occasion.

Official Title

A Phase 1/2 Open-Label Dose Escalation Study to Evaluate the Safety and Efficacy of AGTC-501 (rAAV2tYF-GRK1-RPGR) and a Phase 2 Randomized, Controlled, Masked, Multi-center Study Comparing Two Doses of AGTC-501 in Male Subjects With X-linked Retinitis Pigmentosa Confirmed by a Pathogenic Variant in the RPGR Gene

Conditions

X-linked retinitis pigmentosa

Intervention/Treatment

Biological: rAAV2tYF-GRK1-RPGR

Study Start (Actual)

2018-04-16

Primary Completion (Estimated)

2022-08

Study Completion (Estimated)

2026-08

Enrollment (Estimated)

42

Study Type

Interventional

Phase

Phase 1 Phase 2

Other Study ID Numbers

AGTC-RPGR-001

Study Contact

Name: Serva Health
Phone Number: 855-467-2364
Email: ProviderSupport@scenictrials.com

Study Contact Backup

Name: Jill Dolgin, PharmD
Phone Number: 833-770-2862
Email: advocacy@agtc.com

United States
Florida Locations

Jacksonville, Florida, United States, 32209
Recruiting
University of Florida

Massachusetts Locations

Boston, Massachusetts, United States, 02115
Recruiting
Boston Children's Hospital

Eligibility Criteria
Phase 1/2 Dose Escalation Inclusion Criteria:

- Male subjects between the ages of 6–50 years old with a documented RPGR mutation within exons 1–14 and/or ORF15 from a Clinical Laboratory Improvement Amendments (CLIA)-certified laboratory
- Clinical diagnosis of X-linked retinitis pigmentosa (XLRP)
- Best-corrected visual acuity not better than 78 ETDRS letters (20/32) in the study eye
- Also meet the other requirements of the study as specified in the protocol

Phase 1/2 Dose Escalation Exclusion Criteria:

- Have other known retinal disease mutations or previously received an AAV gene therapy product, as well as being unable or unwilling to meet the requirements of the study

Phase 2 Dose Expansion Inclusion Criteria:

- Males between the ages of 8–50 years old with a clinical diagnosis of XLRP with a confirmed RPGR mutation who also meet the other requirements of the study
- Have at least one documented pathogenic or likely pathogenic variant in the RPGR gene within exons 1–14 and/or ORF15 from Molecular Vision Laboratory (MVL), a CLIA-certified laboratory.
- Both eyes: Have a BCVA no better than 75 letters (20/32) and no worse than 35 letters (20/200) in both eyes based on an ETDRS chart at each screening visit. Pediatric subjects unable to read the ETDRS letters may utilize a tumbling "E" chart for BCVA assessments.

Phase 2 Dose Expansion Exclusion Criteria

- Have other known retinal disease mutations or previously received an AAV gene therapy product, as well as being unable or unwilling to meet the requirements of the study

Ages Eligible for Study
6–50 years (Child, Adult)

Sexes Eligible for Study
Male

Accepts Healthy Volunteers
No

Sponsor
Applied Genetic Technologies Corp

Collaborators
No information provided

Investigators
- Study Director: Matthew Feinsod, MD, Applied Genetics Technologies Corporation

General Publications
No publications available

Recruiting

China

Gene Therapy for Subjects with RPGR Mutation-Associated X-Linked Retinitis Pigmentosa

ClinicalTrials.gov ID NCT05874310

Sponsor: Frontera Therapeutics
Information provided by Frontera Therapeutics (Responsible Party)
Last Update Posted 2023-05-24

Study Overview

Brief Summary
A clinical trial of gene therapy for patients with X-linked retinitis pigmentosa (XLRP).

Official Title
An Open-label, Single-center, Dose-escalation Clinical Study to Evaluate the Safety, Tolerability, and Preliminary Efficacy of Intraocular Administration of FT-002 in Subjects With RPGR Mutation-associated X-linked Retinitis Pigmentosa.

Conditions
X-linked retinitis pigmentosa

Intervention/Treatment
Genetic: FT-002

Study Start (Actual)
2023-02-01

Primary Completion (Estimated)
2023-10-31

Study Completion (Estimated)
2027-11-01

Enrollment (Estimated)
18

Study Type
Interventional

Phase
Early phase 1

Other Study ID Numbers
FT0

Study Contact
Name: Xinyan Li
Phone Number: +86-021-58206061
Email: xinyan.li@fronteratherapeutics.com

Study Contact Backup
Name: Minghui Xue
Phone Number: +86-021-58206061
Email: minghui.xue@fronteratherapeutics.com
China
Beijing Locations

Beijing, Beijing, China, 100142
Recruiting
Peking Union Medical College Hospital

Contact
Ruifang Sui, Professor

Shanghai Locations

Shanghai, Shanghai, China, 200032
Recruiting
Eye & ENT hospital of Fudan university

Contact
Gezhi Xu, Professor

Contact
Jihong Wu, Professor

Eligibility Criteria
Inclusion Criteria
- Subjects that are willing and able to follow study procedures; 2. Males aged 8–45 years old at the time of signing the Informed Consent Form; 3. Subjects who are confirmed with variants of RPGR

Exclusion Criteria
- Have other retinal degenerative diseases, such as retinal degeneration caused by other known inherited retinal disease gene variants or previously received a gene therapy product.

Ages Eligible for Study
8–45 years (Child, Adult)

Sexes Eligible for Study
Male

Accepts Healthy Volunteers
No

Sponsor
Frontera therapeutics

Collaborators
- Eye & ENT Hospital of Fudan University
- Peking Union Medical College Hospital
- Henan Provincial People's Hospital

Investigators
- Principal Investigator: Gezhi Xu, Eye & ENT Hospital of Fudan University
- Principal Investigator: Ruifang Sui, Peking Union Medical College Hospital

General Publications
No publications available

Chapter 11
Not Yet Recruiting Gene Therapy Studies

United States

A Clinical Trial Evaluating the Safety and Efficacy of a Single Subretinal Injection of AGTC-501 in Participants with X-Linked Retinitis Pigmentosa Caused by RPGR Mutations

ClinicalTrials.gov ID NCT04850118

Sponsor Applied Genetic Technologies Corp.
Information provided by Applied Genetic Technologies Corp (Responsible Party).
Last Update Posted on 2021-05-21.

Brief Summary
This study will evaluate and compare the safety, efficacy, and tolerability of two doses of a recombinant adeno-associated virus vector (AGTC-501) to an untreated control group in male patients with X-linked retinitis pigmentosa caused by RPGR mutations.

Detailed Description
This Phase 2/3 study is a randomized, controlled, masked, multicenter study, evaluating and comparing two doses of AGTC-501 to an untreated control group. A single subretinal injection of AGTC-501 Dose 1 (low dose) or Dose 2 (high dose) will be administered in subjects in two treatment groups (N = ~42), while subjects in the untreated control group (N = ~21) will be followed and evaluated up to Month 12, after which they will be eligible to receive treatment with AGTC-501 Dose 2.

Approximately 63 eligible male subjects between 8 and 50 years of age (inclusive) will be randomized in a 1:1:1 ratio to 1 of 3 groups (low dose, high dose, and untreated control).

J. N. Weiss, *Clinical Trials in Retinitis Pigmentosa Treatment*,
https://doi.org/10.1007/978-3-031-58799-3_11

Official Title

A Phase 2/3, Randomized, Controlled, Masked, Multi-center Study to Evaluate the Efficacy, Safety, and Tolerability of Two Doses of AGTC-501, a Recombinant Adeno-associated Virus Vector Expressing RPGR (rAAV2tYF-GRK1-RPGR), Compared to an Untreated Control Group in Male Subjects With X-linked Retinitis Pigmentosa Confirmed by a Pathogenic Variant in the RPGR Gene

Conditions

X-linked retinitis pigmentosa

Intervention/Treatment

Biological: rAAV2tYF-GRK1-hRPGRco

Study Start (Estimated)

2021–08

Primary Completion (Estimated)

2024–01

Study Completion (Estimated)

2029–03

Enrollment (Estimated)

63

Study Type

Interventional

Phase

Phase 2 Phase 3

Other Study ID Numbers

AGTC-RPGR-002

Study Contact

Name: Serva Health
Phone Number: 855–467-2364
Email: ProviderSupport@scenictrials.com
No location data

Eligibility Criteria
Inclusion Criteria

- Males between the ages of 8 and 50 years old with a clinical diagnosis of XLRP with a confirmed RPGR mutation who also meet the other requirements of the study.
- Have at least one documented pathogenic or likely pathogenic variant in the RPGR gene within exons 1–14 and/or ORF15.
- Have a BCVA no better than 75 letters (20/32) and no worse than 35 letters (20/200) in the study eye based on an Early Treatment of Diabetic Retinopathy Study (ETDRS) chart at each screening visit.

Exclusion Criteria

- Have other known retinal disease mutations or previously received an AAV gene therapy product, as well as being unable or unwilling to meet the requirements of the study.

Ages Eligible for Study
8–50 years (Child, Adult)

Sexes Eligible for Study
Male

Accepts Healthy Volunteers
No

Design Details
Primary purpose: Treatment
Allocation: Randomized
Interventional model: Parallel assignment
Interventional model description: Subjects are randomized in a 1:1:1 ratio to 1 of 3 groups (low dose, high dose, and untreated). After 12 months, subjects in the untreated group are eligible to receive the high dose of AGTC-501.
Masking: Quadruple (Participant Care Provider Investigator Outcomes Assessor)
Masking description: For groups 1 and 2 (AGTC-501 dosing groups), both the subjects and the investigators are masked to dose assignment, and only the unmasked staff who prepare the dose are unmasked to the subject's dose assignment. Due to the need to perform the subretinal injection to administer the study drug, both subjects and investigators will know whether the subject was assigned to a treatment group or to the control group. To minimize bias of the treated and control study eye evaluations, starting at Month 3, microperimetry, mobility testing, and BCVA assessments will be conducted by appropriately qualified masked evaluators who do not know whether the subject underwent surgery. Subjects will be instructed not to disclose whether they had surgery to the examiner administering the test.

Arms and interventions

Participant group/arm	Intervention/treatment
Active comparator: Group 1: Low dose Male subjects 8–50 years of age treated by subretinal injection with the low dose of AGTC-501	Biological: rAAV2tYF-GRK1-hRPGRco • Adeno-associated virus vector expressing a human RPGR gene • Other names: – AGTC-501
Active comparator: Group 2: High dose Male subjects 8–50 years of age treated by subretinal injection with the high dose of AGTC-501	Biological: rAAV2tYF-GRK1-hRPGRco • Adeno-associated virus vector expressing a human RPGR gene • Other names: – AGTC-501

Other: Group 3: Control Male subjects 8–50 years of age in the untreated control group. Subjects randomized to the untreated control group will be followed for a minimum of 12 months. After this time, they will be treated by subretinal injection with the high dose of AGTC-501	Biological: rAAV2tYF-GRK1-hRPGRco • Adeno-associated virus vector expressing a human RPGR gene • Other names: – AGTC-501

Primary outcome measures

Outcome measure	Measure description	Time frame
The difference in the proportion of responding eyes between treated and control eyes in low-dose group and high-dose group		Day 0—month 12

Secondary outcome measures

Outcome measure	Measure description	Time frame
– Proportion of responding eyes in treated study eyes in the low-dose group and high-dose group versus untreated control eyes, as measured by mobility test score change		Day 0—month 12
– Proportion of responding eyes in treated eyes versus control eyes in the low-dose and high-dose group measured by visual function assessments		Day 0—month 12
– Difference in mean change from baseline in visual acuity in treated eyes versus control eyes in the low-dose and high-dose groups		Day 0—month 12
– Difference in mean change from baseline in the EZ area, as measured by SD-OCT, in treated study eyes in the low-dose group and high-dose group versus untreated control study eyes		Day 0—month 12
Changes from baseline in quality of life questionnaire responses		Day 0—month 12

Other outcome measures

Outcome measure	Measure description	Time frame
Number and proportion of treatment-emergent adverse events		Day 0—year 5
Number and proportion of participants experiencing abnormal clinically relevant hematology or clinical chemistry parameters		Day 0—year 5

Sponsor
Applied Genetic Technologies Corp

Collaborators
No information provided

Investigators
- Study Director: Matthew Feinsod, MD, Applied Genetic Technologies Corporation

General Publications
No publications available

Chapter 12
Active, Not Recruiting Gene Therapy Studies

United States

RST-001 Phase I/II Trial for Advanced Retinitis Pigmentosa

ClinicalTrials.gov ID NCT02556736

Sponsor AbbVie
Information provided by AbbVie (Responsible Party)
Last Update Posted 2022-10-06

Brief Summary
Currently enrolling a total of 12 patients for Phase 2a of the study: six patients must have VA of no-better-than hand motion in the study eye, and six patients must have VA in the study eye to range from no-worse-than count fingers to 20/200 vision.

Official Title
Phase I/IIa, Open-Label, Dose-Escalation Study of Safety and Tolerability of Intravitreal RST-001 in Patients with Advanced Retinitis Pigmentosa (RP).

Conditions
Advanced Retinitis Pigmentosa

Study Type
Interventional

Enrollment (Actual)
14

Intervention/Treatment
Drug: RST-001

J. N. Weiss, *Clinical Trials in Retinitis Pigmentosa Treatment*,
https://doi.org/10.1007/978-3-031-58799-3_12

Phase
Phase 1 Phase 2

Other Study ID Numbers
RST-001-CP-0001

Study Start (Actual)
2015-12-14

Primary Completion (Actual)
2020-06-01

Study Completion (Estimated)
2024-09-02

United States
California Locations

San Francisco, California, United States, 94143
University of California, San Francisco—Dept. of Ophthalmology

North Carolina Locations

Durham, North Carolina, United States, 27710
Duke Eye Center

Ohio Locations

Cincinnati, Ohio, United States, 45242
Cincinnati Eye Institute

Eligibility Criteria
Ages Eligible for Study
18 years and older (Adult, Older Adult)

Accepts Healthy Volunteer
No

Sexes Eligible for Study
All

Description

Inclusion Criteria
- Participants must meet all of the following criteria.
  - Age > = 18 years.
  - Signed and dated written informed consent obtained from the patient.
  - Ability to comply with testing and all protocol tests.

Exclusion Criteria

- Any one of the following will exclude patients from being enrolled into the study:
  - Unable or unwilling to meet requirements of the study.
  - Participation in a clinical study (ocular or nonocular) with an investigational drug, agent or therapy in the past 6 months.

Design Details

Primary Purpose: Treatment
Allocation: N/A
Interventional Model: Single Group Assignment
Masking: None (Open Label)

Arms and interventions

Participant group/arm	Intervention/treatment
Experimental: Group 1 Single intravitreal injection of RST-001	Drug: RST-001 • RST-001 is a gene therapeutic delivered by intravitreal injection

Primary outcome measures

Outcome measure	Measure description	Time frame
Number of participants with any grade 3 or greater adverse event (AE) considered related to RST-001	The U.S. Dept. of Health and Human Services' common terminology criteria for adverse events grades AEs from 1 (mild) to 5 (death related to AE) Grade 3 is defined as "severe or medically significant but not immediately life-threatening; hospitalization or prolongation of hospitalization indicated; disabling; limiting self-care activities of daily living (ADL)	Baseline (day 1) to 6 months

Sponsor

AbbVie

Collaborators

No information provided

Investigators

Study Director: Hanh Badger, PharmD, Allergan

General Publications

No publications available.

Results

- Outcome measures
  - Number of participants with any grade 3 or greater adverse event (AE) considered related to RST-001.

Type: Primary | Time Frame: Baseline (Day 1) to 6 Months

Description	The U.S. Dept. of Health and Human Services' Common Terminology Criteria for Adverse Events grades AEs from 1 (Mild) to 5 (Death related to AE) Grade 3 is defined as Severe or medically significant but not immediately life-threatening; hospitalization or prolongation of hospitalization indicated; disabling; limiting self-care Activities of Daily Living (ADL)
Time frame	Baseline (day 1) to 6 months
Analysis population description	[Not specified]

Arm/group title	RST-001
Arm/group description	Single intravitreal injection of RST-001
Overall number of participants analyzed	14
Measure type: number	unit of measure: participants	0

Adverse events.
Time frame.

Adverse event data was collected from the screening visit (up to 45 days prior to study drug administration) up to 12 months after drug administration.

Adverse Event Reporting Description
Adverse event data presented includes all adverse events with an onset date on or after the date of drug administration.

Arm/group title	RST-001
Arm/group description	Single intravitreal injection of RST-001
All-cause mortality	
Arm/group title	RST-001
	Affected/at risk (%)
Total	0/14 (0.00%)
Serious adverse events	
Arm/group title	RST-001
	Affected/at risk (%)
Total	0/14 (0.00%)
Other (not including serious) adverse events	
5% Frequency threshold for reporting other adverse events	
Arm/group title	RST-001
	Affected/at risk (%)
Total	9/14 (64.29%)

Eye disorders	
Anterior chamber cell[a,b]	1/14 (7.14%)
Blepharitis[a,b]	1/14 (7.14%)
Conjunctival haemorrhage[a,b]	1/14 (7.14%)
Eye discharge[a,b]	1/14 (7.14%)
Eye irritation[a,b]	1/14 (7.14%)
Eye pain[a,b]	1/14 (7.14%)
Iritis[a,b]	1/14 (7.14%)
Retinal haemorrhage[a,b]	1/14 (7.14%)
Vitreal cells[a,b]	1/14 (7.14%)
Vitreous detachment[a,b]	1/14 (7.14%)
Vitritis[a,b]	1/14 (7.14%)
Gastrointestinal disorders	
Intestinal obstruction[a,b]	1/14 (7.14%)
General disorders	
Swelling[a,b]	1/14 (7.14%)
Infections and infestations	
Ear infection[a,b]	1/14 (7.14%)
Oral fungal infection[a,b]	1/14 (7.14%)
Sialoadenitis[a,b]	1/14 (7.14%)
Tooth infection[a,b]	1/14 (7.14%)
Injury, poisoning and procedural complications	
Fall[a,b]	1/14 (7.14%)
Post-procedural haemorrhage[a,b]	1/14 (7.14%)
Post-traumatic pain[a,b]	1/14 (7.14%)
Investigations	
Intraocular pressure increased[a,b]	3/14 (21.43%)
Metabolism and nutrition disorders	
Hyperkalaemia[a,b]	1/14 (7.14%)
Musculoskeletal and connective tissue disorders	
Arthralgia[a,b]	1/14 (7.14%)
Musculoskeletal chest pain[a,b]	1/14 (7.14%)
Neck pain[a,b]	1/14 (7.14%)
Neoplasms benign, malignant, and unspecified (incl cysts and polyps)	
Benign neoplasm of eyelid[a,b]	1/14 (7.14%)
Nervous system disorders	
Cerebrospinal fluid leakage[a,b]	1/14 (7.14%)
Optic neuritis[a,b]	1/14 (7.14%)
Product issues	
Device dislocation[a,b]	1/14 (7.14%)
Renal and urinary disorders	
Pollakiuria[a,b]	1/14 (7.14%)

[a]Indicates events were collected by systematic assessment
[b]Term from vocabulary, MedDRA 23.0

Sponsor
AbbVie.

Collaborators
No information provided.

Investigators
Study Director: Hanh Badger, PharmD, Allergan.

Publications About Study Results
No publications available.

United States

2.4D-125 in Patients with X-Linked Retinitis Pigmentosa (XLRP)

ClinicalTrials.gov ID NCT04517149

Sponsor 4D Molecular Therapeutics
Information provided by 4D Molecular Therapeutics (Responsible Party)
Last Update Posted 2023-07-28

Study Overview

Brief Summary
This is a Phase 1/2 multicenter study with two parallel parts: an observational natural history cohort and an open-label, prospective interventional trial in males with nonsyndromic X-linked retinitis pigmentosa (XLRP) due to mutations in the gene encoding retinitis pigmentosa GTPase regulator (RPGR).

Detailed Description
This Phase 1/2 study will gather data in an observational phase Natural History Cohort to further characterize and evaluate natural disease progression in male patients with genetically-confirmed X-linked retinitis pigmentosa (XLRP) caused by mutations in the gene encoding retinitis pigmentosa GTPase regulator (RPGR). The study will also evaluate the safety and tolerability, as assessed by frequency and severity of ocular and systemic adverse events, as well as preliminary clinical efficacy of a single intravitreal (IVT) injection of 4D-125 at two dose levels in this patient population in one or both eyes (the contralateral eye dose provided the subject is eligible and provides consent).

4D-125 has been developed as a gene replacement therapy for XLRP. After receiving 4D-125, patients will be followed for 24 months with continued safety follow-up and 36 additional months of long-term follow-up. Secondary endpoints will assess preliminary efficacy measures over time after 4D-125 administration.

Official Title
An Open-label, Phase 1/2 Trial of Gene Therapy 4D-125 in Males with X-linked Retinitis Pigmentosa (XLRP) Caused by Mutations in the RPGR Gene.

Conditions
X-Linked Retinitis Pigmentosa

Intervention/Treatment
Biological: 4D-125 IVT Injection
Other: Observational

Study Start (Actual)
2020-06-09

Primary Completion (Estimated)
2026–06

Study Completion (Estimated)
2029–05

Enrollment (Actual)
21

Study Type
Interventional

Phase
Phase 1 Phase 2

Other Study ID Numbers
4D-125-C001

United States
Colorado Locations

Aurora, Colorado, United States, 80045
University of Colorado

Florida Locations

Gainesville, Florida, United States, 32607
Vitreo Retinal Associates

Michigan Locations

Ann Arbor, Michigan, United States, 48105
University of Michigan Kellogg Eye Center

New York Locations

New York, New York, United States, 10032
Columbia University Medical Center/Edward Harkness Eye Institute

North Carolina Locations

Durham, North Carolina, United States, 27710
Duke University Eye Center/Dept. of Ophthalmology

Oregon Locations

Portland, Oregon, United States, 97239
Casey Eye Institute, Oregon Health and Science University

Texas Locations

Dallas, Texas, United States, 75231
Retina Foundation of the Southwest

Eligibility Criteria

- Natural History Key Inclusion Criteria:
  - Male, ≥ 6 years of age at the time of informed consent
  - Hemizygous nonsyndromic RPGR mutation confirmed by genetic testing

Interventional Key Inclusion Criteria

- Male, ≥12 years of age
- Hemizygous nonsyndromic RPGR mutation confirmed by genetic testing
- Phase 1 Dose Exploration: At least one eye amenable to IVT injection and BCVA ≤78 ETDRS letters (~20/32) and ≥34 ETDRS letters (~20/200)
- Phase 2 Dose Expansion: At least one eye amenable to IVT injection and both eyes must have BCVA ≥34 ETDRS letters (~20/200)

Key Exclusion Criteria (All Cohorts)

- Patient has previously received any AAV treatment
- Preexisting eye conditions or surgical complications that would preclude participation in an interventional clinical trial or interfere with the interpretation of study endpoints

Ages Eligible for Study
12 years and older (Child, Adult, Older Adult)

Sexes Eligible for Study
Male

Accepts Healthy Volunteers
No

Design Details
Primary Purpose: Treatment
Allocation: Nonrandomized
Interventional Model: Sequential Assignment
Interventional Model Description: In Phase 1, up to 2 dose exploration cohorts will be enrolled; each cohort will initially recruit up to three patients to receive a single uniocular IVT injection of 4D-125 in a standard 3 + 3 design. The cohort will be expanded in the event of a dose limiting toxicity (DLT). Any cohort may

be expanded by an additional three subjects (to a maximum of 12 patients) to provide additional safety information and/or to confirm the selected dose for expansion. Once the dose level has been selected, the Phase 2 Dose Expansion Cohort will be opened to dose an additional 6–12 adult patients, and includes a pediatric subpopulation of up to six patients. For adult participants only, the contralateral eye may also be dosed with 4D-125 as a single dose, IVT injection provided the subject is eligible and provides consent.

Masking: None (Open Label)

Arms and interventions

Participant group/arm	Intervention/treatment
Experimental: 4D-125 Dose Exploration Dose 1 and Dose 2 4D-125 will be administered at the assigned dose level as a single dose, IVT injection on day 1. The contralateral eye may also be dosed with 4D-125 as a single dose, IVT injection provided the subject is eligible and provides consent	Biological: 4D-125 IVT Injection • 4D-125 drug product developed for gene therapy, which comprises an AAV capsid variant (4D-R100) carrying a codon-optimized human Retinitis Pigmentosa GTPase Regulator transgene
Experimental: 4D-125 Dose Expansion 4D-125 will be administered at the assigned dose level as a single dose, IVT injection on day 1 in both adults and pediatric participants. For adult participants only, the contralateral eye may also be dosed with 4D-125 as a single dose, IVT injection provided the subject is eligible and provides consent	Biological: 4D-125 IVT Injection • 4D-125 drug product developed for gene therapy, which comprises an AAV capsid variant (4D-R100) carrying a codon-optimized human Retinitis Pigmentosa GTPase Regulator transgene
Other: Observational Natural History	Other: Observational • Natural History

Primary outcome measures

Outcome measure	Measure description	Time frame
Incidence and severity of TEAEs and serious adverse events (SAEs), including clinically significant changes in safety parameters		24 months to 60 months

Sponsor
4D Molecular Therapeutics

Collaborators
No information provided

Investigators
Study Director: Schonmei Lee, MD, 4D Molecular Therapeutics

General Publications
No publications available.

Germany

PDE6A Gene Therapy for Retinitis Pigmentosa (Pigment)

ClinicalTrials.gov ID NCT04611503

Sponsor STZ eyetrial
Information provided by STZ eyetrial (Responsible Party)
Last Update Posted 2022-12-08

Brief Summary
The PDE6A gene encodes a subunit of the rod phosphodiesterase. The loss of this enzyme function leads to a chronically elevated cGMP level which causes an increased calcium inflow into the cell and thereby the hyperactivation of cell death pathways. The goal of the PIGMENT study is to develop, produce and investigate a recombinant adeno-associated viral (AAV) gene transfer vector for the curative therapy of PDE6A-linked retinitis pigmentosa in patients, in order to counteract their disease progression and to stop further impairment of visual function. The vector is given with a single subretinal injection.

Detailed Description
"PIGMENT - Subretinal PDE6A gene therapy for retinitis pigmentosa" is an open monocenter, phase I/IIa trial with fellow-eye comparison.

The study begins with a detailed preliminary examination (Screening), comprises a total of 13 visits and ends after 1 year. In between, after the gene therapy injection (injection of the vector under the retina with one of four doses), regular controls are carried out at the Center for Ophthalmology Tübingen. Monitoring will be continued after the first year, once a year two, three, four, and five years after the injection. The study will take place exclusively at the Center for Ophthalmology in Tübingen and involves nine patients.

All patients participating in this study receive treatment, i.e., there is no placebo or sham treatment group. A 30-day safety distance is maintained between each patient and each group. An independent committee will decide, after each injection of three patients, which dose the following three patients will receive.

Patients can benefit from the treatment by slowing or stopping the loss of the rods and allowing them to function to a certain extent. Therefore, a possible benefit for patients may be that the vision problems will be improved by gene therapy. Such improvements could improve the overall quality of life and well-being. However, as no experience with gene therapy for retinitis pigmentosa in humans has yet been gained, we cannot promise any improvement. Within the scope of this study, patients will be given particularly intensive care and psychological support will also be offered in order to do everything for the patient's well-being and health during the study.

Time Schedule: Start of trial Q3/2019 (FPFV), end of recruitment Q3/2020, end of trial Q4/2025 (LPLV), duration of trial per patient: 1 year with 4 years of follow-up. The final study report will be prepared after completion of the 4 year follow-up period (5 years after treatment).

Official Title
PIGMENT—PDE6A Gene Therapy for Retinitis Pigmentosa.

Conditions
Retinitis Pigmentosa

Intervention/Treatment
Drug: subretinal injection of rAAV.hPDE6A

Study Start (Actual)
2019-09-24

Primary Completion (Estimated)
2023–07

Study Completion (Estimated)
2027–07

Enrollment (Actual)
9

Study Type
Interventional

Phase
Phase 1 Phase 2

Other Study ID Numbers
RDC-PDE6A-01

Germany

Tuebingen, Germany, 72076
Universitätsklinikum Tübingen, Department für Augenheilkunde

Eligibility Criteria
Inclusion Criteria
- Clinical diagnosis of retinitis pigmentosa
- Confirmed mutation in PDE6A gene
- $\geq$ 18 years of age
- Visual acuity $\geq$20/400
- No infection with Human Immunodeficiency Virus (HIV)
- Negative pregnancy test in women with childbearing potential (a woman who is 2 years postmenopausal or surgically sterile is not considered to be of childbearing potential)
- Male patients must agree to use condoms during the first 6 months post treatment
- Female patients of childbearing potential must agree to use an effective method of birth control during the first 6 months post treatment
- Ability to understand and willingness to consent to study protocol

Exclusion Criteria

- Ocular (study eye & fellow eye)
  - Additional interfering ocular conditions with impact on study results (e.g., ocular opacity and advanced cataract, uveitis and amblyopia)
  - Recent (6 months) ocular surgery, intravitreal or subretinal implantation of a medical device
  - Disease causing mutations in another known retinitis pigmentosa gene
  - Ocular infection with herpes simplex virus in medical history
  - History of ocular malignancies
  - Disorders of the internal retina (e.g., retinal detachment in the patient's history)
  - Glaucoma defined as damage of the optic nerve
  - Vascular retinal occlusion
  - Diabetic patients suffering from retinopathy and/or macula edema
  - Any other retinopathy due to other diseases, e.g., (but not limited to) arterial hypertension, trauma or acquired inflammatory diseases (uveitis serology), contraindication to pharmacological mydriasis (e.g., history of angle block glaucoma)
  - Absence of visual function on the contralateral eye Systemic
  - Systemic conditions (e.g., coronary heart disease, autoimmune disorders) which may affect study participation or outcome measures
  - History of poorly controlled diabetes mellitus type 1 or type 2
  - Systemic illness or medically relevant abnormal laboratory values in blood analysis including renal and hepatic functions at inclusion
  - Patients treated with oral corticoids within 14 days prior inclusion
  - Current or recent participation in other study/or administration of biologic agent within the last 3 months
  - Known sensitivity to any compound used in the study
  - Contraindications to systemic immunosuppression
  - Contraindications in view of the planned surgery (e.g., but not limited to anaemia Hb < 10 g/dl, coagulopathy with PT/PTT >1.5-fold upper limit, hypertension with values above 180 mmHg systolic and 110 mmHg diastolic) including intolerance and contraindications to general anesthesia
  - Intolerance to contrast agents used for diagnostic methods like angiography with fluoresceine or indocyanine green (e.g., but not limited to hyperthyroidism, hepatic insufficiency)
  - Subject/partner of childbearing potential unwilling to use adequate contraception for 4 months
  - Nursing or pregnant women
  - Any other cause that, in the investigator's opinion, renders potential subjects not suitable for the study

Ages Eligible for Study
18 years and older (Adult, Older Adult)

Sexes Eligible for Study
All

Accepts Healthy Volunteers
No

Design Details
Primary Purpose: Treatment
Allocation: N/A
Interventional Model: Sequential Assignment
Masking: None (Open Label)

Arms and interventions

Participant group/ arm	Intervention/treatment
Experimental: Subretinal injection of rAAV.hPDE6A Single subretinal injection of rAAV.hPDE6A	Drug: subretinal injection of rAAV.hPDE6A • The first three patients (C1) will receive the intermediate dose 1×1010 vg. After injection of the third patient of C1, the DMC will give a go/no go decision. If 'nogo', a lower dose (5 × 109 vg) will be given to the next group of three patients (C2). The DMC will give a go/no go decision. In case of a "go" decision, three further patients (C3) will be treated with the same dose. In the case of a no-go decision, the next dose will be the minimal dose 1 × 109 vg. In case of a 'go' decision of the DMC after the third patient, the next three patients will receive a subretinal injection of vector at the highest dose 5 × 1010 vg. The DMC will give a go/no go decision after review of all safety data available at D30 of cohort 2. If safety data is considered favourably by the DMC, then three further patients (cohort 3) will be treated with the same dose (5 × 1010 vg). Should any safety concerns arise, the last three patients (cohort 3) will receive the intermediate dose (1 × 1010 vg) • Other names – Gene therapy

Primary outcome measures

Outcome measure	Measure description	Time frame
Slit lamp examination	To determine possibly occurring ocular inflammation and to observe if there are any treatment effects	1 year +4 years follow-up
Fundus biomicroscopy to determine possibly occurring ocular inflammation and to observe if there are any treatment effects	To determine possibly occurring ocular inflammation and to observe if there are any treatment effects	1 year +4 years follow-up
Angiography	To determine possibly occurring ocular inflammation and to observe if there are any treatment effects	1 year +4 years follow-up

Secondary outcome measures

Outcome measure	Measure description	Time frame
Visual acuity	To determine any therapy effects concerning visual acuity	1 year +4 years follow-up
Contrast sensitivity	To determine any therapy effects concerning the contrast sensitivity	1 year +4 years follow-up
Visual field	To determine any therapy effects concerning the visual field	1 year +4 years follow-up
Colour vision	To determine any therapy effects concerning colour vision	1 year +4 years follow-up
Pupillography	To determine any therapy effects concerning pupil reaction	1 year +4 years follow-up
Electrophysiology	To determine any therapy effects concerning the electrophysiology	1 year +4 years follow-up

Sponsor
STZ eyetrial

Collaborators
No information provided

Investigators
- Principal Investigator: Dominik Fischer, Prof., University Hospital Tuebingen

General Publications
No publications available.

Sweden

A First-In-Human, Proof of Concept Study of CPK850 in Patients with RLBP1 Retinitis Pigmentosa

ClinicalTrials.gov ID NCT03374657

Sponsor: Novartis Pharmaceuticals
Information provided by Novartis Pharmaceuticals (Responsible Party)
Last update posted on 2023-07-13

Brief Summary
The purpose of this first-in-human study is to explore the maximum tolerated dose (MTD) of CPK850 as determined by the single ascending dose ranging portion of the study. This study will also evaluate the safety and potential efficacy of CPK850 on improving visual function in patients with decreased visual function from RLBP1 retinitis pigmentosa due to biallelic mutations in the RLBP1 gene.

Detailed Description
This study will potentially include five cohorts with a minimum of three patients per cohort, with an optional cohort of up to six patients. This trial design uses a staggered patient enrollment with continuous data reviews to limit as much unforeseen risk as possible prior to enrolling each patient in each cohort or initiating another cohort. Only one eye (designated as the study or treated eye) will be dosed per patient. Each patient will be followed for 5 years after the subretinal injection of CPK850.

Official Title
An Open-label First-in-human Single Ascending Dose Study to Explore Safety, Tolerability, and Efficacy of Subretinal Administration of CPK850 Gene Therapy in Patients with Retinitis Pigmentosa due to Mutations in the Retinaldehyde Binding Protein 1 (RLBP1) Gene

Conditions
Retinitis Pigmentosa

Intervention/Treatment
Biological: CPK850

Study Start (Actual)
2018-08-22

Primary Completion (Estimated)
2026-05-11

Study Completion (Estimated)
2026-05-11

Enrollment (Actual)
12

Study Type
Interventional

Phase
Phase 1 Phase 2

Other Study ID Numbers
CCPK850X2202
2016–002696-10 (EudraCT Number)

Sweden

Stockholm, Sweden, SE-112 82
Novartis Investigative Site

Eligibility Criteria
Inclusion Criteria

- Male and female patients aged 18 to 70 years inclusive.
- The visual acuity in the study eye at the screening 1 visit should be no better than 60 ETDRS letters.
- Clinical diagnosis of Bothnia dystrophy, Newfoundland rod-cone dystrophy or other progressive retinitis pigmentosa phenotype with mutations in the RLBP1 gene verified by genetic testing.
- Visible photoreceptor (outer nuclear) and Retinal Pigment Epithelium (RPE) layers on standard OCT scan in the study eye at the screening 1 visit.

Exclusion Criteria

- History of hypersensitivity to the study drug or to drugs of similar classes or to any of the medications required in the perioperative period.
- Preexisting eye conditions that would preclude the planned surgery or interfere with the interpretation of study endpoints.
- Any contraindication to the planned surgery or anesthesia as determined by the treating physician (surgeon, anesthesiologist, internist, or designee).
- Women who are pregnant, or lactating or women of childbearing potential, defined as all women physiologically capable of becoming pregnant, unless they are using highly effective methods of contraception during dosing and for 2 months after treatment.

Ages Eligible for Study
18 years to 70 years (Adult, Older Adult)

Sexes Eligible for Study
All

Accepts Healthy Volunteers
No

Design Details
Primary Purpose: Treatment
Allocation: Nonrandomized
Interventional Model: Single Group Assignment
Interventional Model Description: This is a nonconfirmatory, open-label single ascending dose gene replacement-therapy study to assess safety, tolerability, and efficacy of CPK850 in patients with RLBP1 retinitis pigmentosa due to biallelic mutations in the RLBP1 gene. The trial design uses a staggered patient enrollment.
Masking: Single (Outcomes Assessor)
Masking Description:
This is a partially masked study. The patients will not be masked. The treating physicians and personnel at the surgical location (surgeons, anesthesiologist, operating room personnel, and others) will not be masked.

At the clinical sites, there will be an unmasked ophthalmologist. The remaining assessors at the clinical sites (ophthalmologist, study nurse, ophthalmic technician, etc.) doing the ophthalmic examinations should be masked to the study (treated) eye.

The following unmasked sponsor roles are required for this study:

Sponsor clinical staff required to assist in the management and resupply of investigational drug product.

The independent committee assessing unmasked interim results and the independent analysis team.

All other sponsor staff will stay masked to treatment assignments.

Arms and interventions

Participant group/arm	Intervention/treatment
Experimental: CPK Dose 1 (lowest dose) CPK850, one subretinal injection to the study eye	Biological: CPK850 • In one of five dose levels administered via subretinal injection under anesthesia
Experimental: CPK Dose 2 (next lowest dose) CPK850, one subretinal injection to the study eye	Biological: CPK850 • In one of five dose levels administered via subretinal injection under anesthesia
Experimental: CPK Dose 3 (third lowest dose) CPK850, one subretinal injection to the study eye	Biological: CPK850 • In one of five dose levels administered via subretinal injection under anesthesia
Experimental: CPK Dose 4 (next to highest dose) CPK850, one subretinal injection to the study eye	Biological: CPK850 • In one of five dose levels administered via subretinal injection under anesthesia
Experimental: CPK Dose 5 (highest dose) CPK850, one subretinal injection to the study eye	Biological: CPK850 • In one of five dose levels administered via subretinal injection under anesthesia

Primary outcome measures

Outcome measure	Measure description	Time frame
Number of participants with adverse events (AEs), serious adverse events (SAEs) and deaths	Safety events	Up to year 5
Number of responders in dark adaptation	A patient is considered a responder if sensitivity recovery values at 1 h postbleach are observed to be outside of the patient's prediction interval at ≥2 consecutive posttreatment visits within 1 year after treatment	Screening/baseline up to year 1

Secondary outcome measures

Outcome measure	Measure description	Time frame
Number of patients with recovery of the cone system	Cone recovery during dark adaptation	Screening/baseline up to year 1
Number of patients with improvement in rod function in the treated eye vs the untreated eye	Rod function during dark adaptation	Screening/baseline up to year 1
Change from screening/baseline in visual field perimetry mean deviation	Assessed using automated static perimetry	Screening/baseline up to year 1
Change from screening/baseline in Total contrast sensitivity score	Contrast sensitivity (i.e., the ability to detect relatively dim objects) will be assessed	Screening/baseline up to year 1
Change from screening/baseline in light-adapted microperimetry sensitivity	Assessed using standard microperimetry equipment	Screening/baseline up to year 1
Change from screening/baseline in the local electrical activity of the retina	Assessed using a system designed to record multifocal electroretinogram (ERG) responses from a number of locations at one time	Screening/baseline up to year 1
Change from screening/baseline in the electrical activity of the retina	Assessed using a system designed to record full-field electroretinogram (ERG) responses with Ganzfeld stimulation.	Screening/baseline up to year 1
Change from screening/baseline in Reading speed	Assessed using standard reading speed charts	Screening/baseline up to year 1
Change from screening/baseline in eye dominance	Dominant eye for viewing targets at distance	Screening/baseline up to year 1
Change from screening/baseline in change from baseline in mobility test scores	Assessed using a system designed to measure the ability to navigate obstacles in a maze-like environment under varying light conditions	Screening/baseline up to year 1
Change from screening/baseline in the National Eye Institute—Visual function questionnaire 25 (NEI-VFQ 25) composite score	Questionnaire completed by the participant to measure the influence of visual impairment on quality of life	Screening/baseline up to year 1
Change from screening/baseline in the low luminance questionnaire (LLQ) responses	Questionnaire completed by the participant to assess visual problems under low luminance conditions, including nighttime	Screening/baseline up to year 1

Sponsor
Novartis Pharmaceuticals

Collaborators
No information provided

Investigators
- Study Director: Novartis Pharmaceuticals, Novartis Pharmaceuticals

General Publications
No publications available.

Chapter 13
Enrolling by Invitation Gene Therapy Studies

United States/Canada/Europe

Long-Term Safety and Efficacy Follow-Up of BIIB111 for the Treatment of Choroideremia and BIIB112 for the Treatment of X-Linked Retinitis Pigmentosa (SOLSTICE)

ClinicalTrials.gov ID NCT03584165

Sponsor NightstaRx Ltd., a Biogen Company
Information provided by NightstaRx Ltd., a Biogen Company (Responsible Party)
Last update posted on 2023-05-08

Brief Summary
The objective of the study is to evaluate the long-term safety and efficacy of a subretinal injection of BIIB111 in participants with choroideremia (CHM) who have been previously treated with BIIB111 and who have exited an antecedent study; these treated participants will be compared with untreated control participants who have exited the STAR (NCT03496012) study and BIIB112 in participants with X-linked retinitis pigmentosa (XLRP) who have been previously treated with BIIB112 and who have exited an antecedent study.

Detailed Description
This study was previously posted by NightstaRx Ltd. In October 2020, sponsorship of the trial was transferred to Biogen.

Official Title
A Long-term Follow-up Study to Evaluate the Safety and Efficacy of Retinal Gene Therapy in Subjects With Choroideremia Previously Treated With Adeno-Associated Viral Vector Encoding Rab Escort Protein-1 (AAV2-REP1)

J. N. Weiss, *Clinical Trials in Retinitis Pigmentosa Treatment*,
https://doi.org/10.1007/978-3-031-58799-3_13

and in Subjects With X-Linked Retinitis Pigmentosa Previously Treated With Adeno-Associated Viral Vector Encoding RPGR (AAV8-RPGR) in an Antecedent Study.

Conditions
Choroideremia
X-linked retinitis pigmentosa

Intervention/Treatment
Genetic: BIIB111
Genetic: BIIB112

Study Start (Actual)
2018-06-04

Primary Completion (Estimated)
2026-06-04

Study Completion (Estimated)
2026-06-04

Enrollment (Estimated)
330

Study Type
Interventional

Phase
Phase 3

Other Study ID Numbers
273CH201
2017-003104-42 (EudraCT Number)

United States
California Locations

Los Angeles, California, United States, 90095-7065
UCLA—Jules Stein Eye Institute

Florida Locations

Gainesville, Florida, United States, 32607
Vitreo Retinal Associates PA—The Millennium Center

Miami, Florida, United States, 33136
University of Miami

Maryland Locations

Baltimore, Maryland, United States, 21287-0005
Johns Hopkins Hospital

Massachusetts Locations

Boston, Massachusetts, United States, 02114-3002
MEEI Massachusetts Eye and Ear Infirmary

New York Locations

New York, New York, United States, 10032
Columbia University Medical Center

Ohio Locations

Cincinnati, Ohio, United States, 45242-5664
Cincinnati Eye Institute—Blue Ash

Oregon Locations

Portland, Oregon, United States, 97239
OHSU—Casey Eye Institute

Texas Locations

Dallas, Texas, United States, 75231-5080
Retina Foundation of the Southwest

Wisconsin Locations

Madison, Wisconsin, United States, 53705-3644
University of Wisconsin School of Medicine

Brazil

Sao Paulo, Brazil, 04039
Instituto Genetica Ocular

Canada
Alberta Locations

Edmonton, Alberta, Canada, T5H 3V9
The Northern Alberta Clinical Trials and Research Centre

British Columbia Locations

Vancouver, British Columbia, Canada, V5Z 39N
The University of British Columbia—Eye Care Centre

Quebec Locations

Montreal, Quebec, Canada, H4A 3JI
McGill University Health Centre

Denmark

Glostrup, Denmark, 2600
Rigshospitalet-Glostrup, Oejenafdelingen

Finland

Helsinki, Finland, 00290 HUS
Helsinki University Central Hospital (HUCH)

France

Montpellier, France, 34295
CHU Montpellier—Saint Eloi

Paris, France, 75012
Centre Hospitalier National d Ophtalmologie (CHNO) des Quinze-Vingts

Germany

Bonn, Germany, 53127
Universitäts-Augenklinik Bonn

Tübingen, Germany, 72076
Universitats Klinikum Tubingen—Institute for Ophthalmic Research

Netherlands

Nijmegen, Netherlands, 6525 GA
Radboudumc

United Kingdom

London, United Kingdom, EC1V 2PD
Moorfields Eye Hospital

Manchester, United Kingdom, M13 9WL
Manchester Royal Eye Hospital

Oxford, United Kingdom, OX3 9DU
John Radcliffe Hospital

Southampton, United Kingdom, SO16 6YD
Southampton General Hospital

Eligibility Criteria
Key Inclusion Criteria
CHM participants.
Have participated in and exited from an interventional study that investigated the safety and efficacy of a subretinal injection of BIIB111 for CHM.
XLRP participants.
Have received a subretinal injection of BIIB112 for XLRP and have exited an antecedent study.

Key Exclusion Criteria

Participants are not eligible for study participation if they meet the following exclusion criterion.

In the opinion of the investigator and/or the sponsor, it is not in the participant's best interest to participate in the study.

Note: Other protocol defined inclusion/exclusion criteria may apply.

Ages Eligible for Study

18 years and older (Adult, Older Adult)

Sexes Eligible for Study

Male

Accepts Healthy Volunteers

No

Design Details

Primary purpose: Others
Allocation: Nonrandomized
Interventional model: Parallel assignment
Masking: Single (Outcomes Assessor)

Arms and interventions

Participant group/arm	Intervention/treatment
Experimental: BIIB111 Participants previously treated with subretinal injection of BIIB111 in antecedent studies 273CH301 (NCT03496012) and 273CH203 (NCT03507686) will be enrolled. Participants previously treated with this same subretinal injection (rAAV2-REP1) in antecedent studies 20,150,371 (NCT02553135), Pro00028599 (NCT02077361), THOR-TUE-01 (NCT02671539), CHM09/01 (NCT01461213) and REGEN2015 (NCT02407678) will also be invited for enrollment. This is a follow-up study, investigational product was administered in the previous study	Genetic: BIIB111 • Administered as specified in the treatment arm • Other Names: – AAV2-REP1 – rAAV2-REP1
Experimental: BIIB112 Participants previously treated with subretinal injection of BIIB112 in the antecedent study 274RP101 (NCT03116113) will be enrolled. This is a follow-up study, investigational product was administered in the previous study	Genetic: BIIB112 • Administered as specified in the treatment arm • Other Names: – AAV8-RPGR
No intervention: Untreated Untreated participants who served as controls in the antecedent study 273CH301 (NCT03496012), investigating treatment with BIIB111, will be enrolled. This is a follow-up study, participants will not be administered study medication nor receive a sham surgery	

Primary outcome measures

Outcome measure	Measure description	Time frame
Percentage of participants with adverse events (AEs)		Up to 5 years
Ophthalmic examination assessment: Intraocular pressure (IOP)		Up to 5 years
Ophthalmic examination assessment: abnormal slit lamp examination		Up to 5 years
Ophthalmic examination assessment: lens opacity grading		Up to 5 years
Ophthalmic examination assessment: Anterior chamber and vitreous inflammation		Up to 5 years
Ophthalmic examination assessment: indirect ophthalmoscopy		Up to 5 years

Secondary outcome measures

Outcome measure	Measure description	Time frame
Change from baseline in best-corrected visual acuity (BCVA)	BCVA will be assessed for both eyes using the early treatment of diabetic retinopathy study (ETDRS) visual acuity (VA) chart. BCVA test should be performed prior to pupil dilation, and distance refraction should be carried out before BCVA is measured. Initially, letters are read at a distance of 4 meters from the chart. If <20 letters are read at 4 meters, testing at 1 meter should be performed. BCVA is to be reported as number of letters read correctly by the participant using the ETDRS Scale (ranging from 0 to 100 letters) in the study eye. The lower the number of letters read correctly on the eye chart, the worse the vision (or visual acuity). An increase in the number of letters read correctly means that vision has improved	Up to 5 years
Percentage of participants with no decrease from baseline in BCVA or a decrease from baseline in BCVA of <5 ETDRS letters in choroideremia (CHM) participants	BCVA will be assessed for both eyes using the early treatment of diabetic retinopathy study (ETDRS) visual acuity (VA) chart. BCVA test should be performed prior to pupil dilation, and distance refraction should be carried out before BCVA is measured. Initially, letters are read at a distance of 4 meters from the chart. If <20 letters are read at 4 meters, testing at 1 meter should be performed. BCVA is to be reported as number of letters read correctly by the participant using the ETDRS scale (ranging from 0 to 100 letters) in the study eye. The lower the number of letters read correctly on the eye chart, the worse the vision (or visual acuity). An increase in the number of letters read correctly means that vision has improved	Up to 5 years

Percentage of participants with an increase from baseline in BCVA of ≥10 ETDRS letters in CHM participants	BCVA will be assessed for both eyes using the early treatment of diabetic retinopathy study (ETDRS) visual acuity (VA) chart. BCVA test should be performed prior to pupil dilation, and distance refraction should be carried out before BCVA is measured. Initially, letters are read at a distance of 4 meters from the chart. If <20 letters are read at 4 meters, testing at 1 meter should be performed. BCVA is to be reported as number of letters read correctly by the participant using the ETDRS scale (ranging from 0 to 100 letters) in the study eye. The lower the number of letters read correctly on the eye chart, the worse the vision (or visual acuity). An increase in the number of letters read correctly means that vision has improved	Up to 5 years
Percentage of participants with an increase from baseline in BCVA of ≥15 ETDRS letters in CHM participants	BCVA will be assessed for both eyes using the early treatment of diabetic retinopathy study (ETDRS) visual acuity (VA) chart. BCVA test should be performed prior to pupil dilation, and distance refraction should be carried out before BCVA is measured. Initially, letters are read at a distance of 4 meters from the chart. If <20 letters are read at 4 meters, testing at 1 meter should be performed. BCVA is to be reported as number of letters read correctly by the participant using the ETDRS scale (ranging from 0 to 100 letters) in the study eye. The lower the number of letters read correctly on the eye chart, the worse the vision (or visual acuity). An increase in the number of letters read correctly means that vision has improved	Up to 5 years
Assessment of fundus autofluorescence (AF) at each visit	Fundus autofluorescence will be performed on both eyes to assess the change in the area of viable retinal tissue. It will be reported in square millimetres (mm^2).	Up to 5 years
Assessment of fundus photography at each visit	Fundus photography will be performed on both eyes following the dilation of the participant's pupils	Up to 5 years
Assessment of spectral domain optical coherence tomography (SD-OCT) at each visit	SD-OCT will be performed on both eyes to assess the foveal changes and other potential anatomic changes. The measurements were taken after dilation of the participant's pupil and would be reported in micrometres (µm)	Up to 5 years
Assessment of Microperimetry at each visit	Microperimetry will be performed on both eyes to assess changes in retinal sensitivity within the macula. It will be reported in decibels (dB)	Up to 5 years
Change from baseline in 25-item visual function questionnaire (VFQ-25)	VFQ-25 questionnaire measures dimensions of self-reported vision-targeted health status that are most important to persons with eye disease. Total score ranges from 0–100, where a score of 0 represents the worst outcome and 100 represents the best outcome	Up to 5 years
Change from baseline in visual field	The outcome measure will be assessed in BIIB112-treated participants	Up to 5 years

Percentage of participants with an increase from baseline in luminance visual acuity (LLVA) of ≥10 ETDRS letters in BIIB112-treated participants	The LLVA was measured by placing a 2.0-log-unit neutral density filter over the best correction for that eye and having the participant read the normally illuminated ETDRS chart. The assessment was performed prior to dilating the eyes. Initially, letters are read at a distance of 4 metres from the chart. If <20 letters are read at 4 metres, testing at 1 metre should be performed. BCVA is to be reported as number of letters read correctly by the participant.	18 months to 60 months, postday 0 visits
Percentage of participants with an increase from baseline in luminance visual acuity (LLVA) of ≥15 ETDRS letters in BIIB112-treated participants	The LLVA was measured by placing a 2.0-log-unit neutral density filter over the best correction for that eye and having the participant read the normally illuminated ETDRS chart. The assessment was performed prior to dilating the eyes. Initially, letters are read at a distance of 4 metres from the chart. If <20 letters are read at 4 metres, testing at 1 metre should be performed. BCVA is to be reported as number of letters read correctly by the participant	18 months to 60 months, postday 0 visits

Sponsor
NightstaRx Ltd., a Biogen Company

Collaborators
No information provided

Investigators
- Study Director: Medical Director, Biogen

General Publications
No publications available.

Note:
There is a rationale for combining a genetic with a stem cell treatment for optimal visual results.

India

A Long-Term Follow-Up Study in Subjects Who Received vMCO-I Administered Via Intravitreal Injection (EXTEND)

ClinicalTrials.gov ID NCT05921162

Sponsor Nanoscope Therapeutics Inc.
Information provided by Nanoscope Therapeutics Inc. (Responsible Party)
Last Update Posted 2023-08-02

Brief Summary
This study "A Long-Term Follow-up Study in Subjects Who Received an Adeno-Associated Viral Vector Serotype 2 Containing the Multicharacteristic Opsin Gene (vMCO-I) Administered Via Intravitreal Injection" is an observational study and will be conducted following Good Clinical Practice (GCP) - International Conference on Harmonization (ICH) guidelines. Eligible subjects satisfying all inclusion and none of the exclusion criteria will be enrolled. All subject who completed the parent clinical study (NSCT/CT/18/01) will undergo safety and efficacy assessments up to 5 years post study drug injection.

Detailed Description
The observational study population comprises of individuals who received an Adeno-Associated Viral Vector Serotype 2 Containing the Multicharacteristic Opsin Gene (vMCO-I) Administered Via Intravitreal Injection in a parent study.

Enrolled subjects will undergo safety and efficacy assessments for up to 5 years from the vMCO-I administration. At the visits, subjects will have safety and efficacy evaluations. Subjects will have a final visit at 60 months post study drug administration.

Official Title
A Long-Term Follow-up Study in Subjects Who Received an Adeno-Associated Viral Vector Serotype 2 Containing the Multicharacteristic Opsin Gene (vMCO-I) Administered Via Intravitreal Injection.

Conditions
Retinitis pigmentosa
Retinal disease
Retinal degeneration

Intervention/treatment
Biological: Gene Therapy product: vMCO-I

Study Start (Actual)
2023-07-14

Primary Completion (Estimated)
2024–12

Study Completion (Estimated)
2024–12

Enrollment (Estimated)
11

Study Type
Observational

Other Study ID Numbers
NTXMCO-005

India
Odisha Locations

Cuttack, Odisha, India, 753014
JPM Rotary Club of Cuttack Eye Hospital and Research Institute

Eligibility Criteria

Inclusion Criteria

- The subject population includes subjects who received an adeno-associated viral vector serotype 2 Containing the multicharacteristic opsin gene (vMCO-I), administered via intravitreal injection in a parent study.

Exclusion Criteria

- Subjects who will not consent for study.

Study Population

It is expected that a total of 11 study subjects from NSCT/CT/18/01 study will be enrolled. Subjects who meet all the inclusion criteria and for whom none of the exclusion criteria apply will be eligible for enrollment.

Ages Eligible for Study

18 years and older (Adult, Older Adult)

Sexes Eligible for Study

All

Accepts Healthy Volunteers

No

Sampling Method

Nonprobability sample

Sponsor

Nanoscope Therapeutics Inc.

Collaborators

No information provided

Investigators

- Study Director: Samarendra Mohanty, Nanoscope Therapeutics Inc.

General Publications

No publications available.

Part III
Optogenetics

Chapter 14
Active, Not Recruiting Optogenetics Studies

United States

Efficacy and Safety of MCO-010 Optogenetic Therapy in Adults with Retinitis Pigmentosa [RESTORE]

ClinicalTrials.gov ID NCT04945772

Sponsor Nanoscope Therapeutics Inc.
Information provided by Nanoscope Therapeutics Inc. (Responsible Party)
Last update posted on 2023-05-31

Brief Summary
The purpose of the study is to evaluate the safety and efficacy of a single intravitreal injection of virally-carried multicharacteristic opsin (MCO-010).

Detailed Description
This multicenter, randomized, double-masked, sham-controlled, dose-ranging study will evaluate two dose levels of MCO-010 in up to 18 subjects with retinitis pigmentosa (nine per dose). Nine subjects will receive sham injection. Subjects with a confirmed diagnosis of advanced retinitis pigmentosa (RP) based on clinical examination, dilated fundus examination, and genetic testing will be considered for participation in this study. All subjects will continue to be assessed for 52 weeks following treatment with MCO-010.

Official Title
A Phase 2b Randomized, Double-Masked, Sham-Controlled, Study to Evaluate the Efficacy and Safety of Intravitreal Injection of MCO-010 Optogenetic Therapy in Adults With Retinitis Pigmentosa (RESTORE).

J. N. Weiss, *Clinical Trials in Retinitis Pigmentosa Treatment*,
https://doi.org/10.1007/978-3-031-58799-3_14

Conditions
Retinitis Pigmentosa
Retinitis
Retinal Diseases
Eye Diseases
Eye Diseases, Hereditary
Retinal Dystrophies
Retinal Degeneration

Intervention/Treatment
Biological: Gene Therapy Product-MCO-010
Procedure: Sham Injection

Study Start (Actual)
2021-07-13

Primary Completion (Actual)
2023-03-28

Study Completion (Estimated)
2024-03-01

Enrollment (Actual)
27

Study Type
Interventional

Phase
Phase 2

Other Study ID Numbers
NTXMCO-002

United States
California Locations

Beverly Hills, California, United States, 90211
Nanoscope Clinical Site

Florida Locations

Pensacola, Florida, United States, 32503
Nanoscope Clinical Site

North Dakota Locations

Fargo, North Dakota, United States, 58103
Nanoscope Clinical Site

Texas Locations

Houston, Texas, United States, 77030
Nanoscope Clinical Site

McAllen, Texas, United States, 78503
Nanoscope Clinical Site

Puerto Rico

Arecibo, Puerto Rico, 00612
Nanoscope Clinical Site

Eligibility Criteria
Inclusion Criteria

- The subject population includes subjects with advanced RP. Subjects are eligible to be included in the study only if all of the following criteria apply:
  - Age ≥ 18 years.
  - Able to comprehend and give informed consent.
  - Confirmed diagnosis of advanced retinitis pigmentosa (RP) based on clinical examination, dilated fundus examination, and genetic testing.
  - Best-corrected (Freiburg) visual acuity worse than 1.9 LogMAR (Snellen equivalent 20/1600, Count Fingers/ Hand Motion) in the study eye and no better than 1.6 LogMAR (Snellen equivalent 20/800) in the fellow eye during screening.
  - Presence of retinal inner nuclear and nerve fiber layers on optical coherence tomography (OCT) testing in the study eye during screening as determined by the investigator and confirmed by the sponsor or designee.

Exclusion Criteria

- Subjects are excluded from the study if any of the following criteria apply:
  - Prior participation in gene therapy program.
  - Individuals who refuse or are incapable of performing mobility testing or pass the mobility testing at 0.3 or 1 lux as determined by the investigator and confirmed by the sponsor or designee during screening, will be excluded.
  - Presence of an active implantable medical device.
  - Preexisting conditions in the study eye such as glaucoma, diseases affecting the optic nerve causing significant visual field loss, active uveitis, corneal or lenticular opacities.
  - Presence of any complicating systemic diseases such as malignancies whose treatment could affect central nervous system function.
  - Subjects who are positive for syphilis, hepatitis B, C, and human immunodeficiency virus (HIV) will be excluded.
  - Subjects who have undergone ocular surgery in the study eye within 3 months prior to Day 0.
  - Presence of narrow iridocorneal angles contraindicating pupillary dilation in the study eye.
  - Presence of disorders of the ocular media in the study eye which could interfere with visual acuity and other ocular assessments, including OCT, during the study period.

- Presence of vitreomacular adhesion or traction, epiretinal membrane, macular pucker, and macular hole in the study eye, evident by ophthalmoscopy and/or by OCT examinations and assessed by the investigator to significantly affect central vision.
- Current evidence of retinal detachment in the study eye that significantly affects central vision.
- Current use of hydroxychloroquine, chloroquine, or any related retina-toxic compounds.
- Active ocular inflammation or recurrent history of idiopathic or autoimmune associated uveitis.
- Having received retinal prothesis (such as ARGUS-II) or any gene or stem cell therapy (ocular or nonocular).

Ages Eligible for Study
18 years and older (Adult, Older Adult)

Sexes Eligible for Study
All

Accepts Healthy Volunteers
No

Design Details
Primary Purpose: Treatment
Allocation: Randomized
Interventional Model: Sequential Assignment
Interventional Model Description: Following a 1:1:1 block randomization schema, nine subjects will be enrolled in each MCO-010 treatment group, and nine subjects will be enrolled in the sham-controlled group.
Masking: Triple (Participant Investigator Outcomes Assessor)
Masking Description: Treatment assignment will be unknown (or masked) to the study participants, the evaluating physician (noninjecting), outcomes assessor, the sponsor and its agents.

Arms and interventions

Participant group/arm	Intervention/treatment
Experimental: MCO-010-High Dose Participants receive 1.2E11gc/eye of MCO-010	Biological: Gene Therapy Product-MCO-010 • The MCO-010 is an adeno-associated virus serotype 2-based vector carried multicharacteristic opsin (MCO) gene expression cassette
Experimental: MCO-010-Medium Dose Participants receive 0.9E11gc/eye of MCO-010	Biological: Gene Therapy Product-MCO-010 • The MCO-010 is an adeno-associated virus serotype 2-based vector carried multicharacteristic opsin (MCO) gene expression cassette
Sham Comparator: Sham Injection Participants receive sham injection	Procedure: Sham Injection • Sham Injection

Primary outcome measures

Outcome measure	Measure description	Time frame
Efficacy of a single intravitreal injection of multicharacteristic opsin (MCO-010) assessed by Multiluminance Y-Mobility Test	Change from baseline in multiluminance Y-mobility test (MLYMT) score for the study eye at week 52	100 weeks

Secondary outcome measures

Outcome measure	Measure description	Time frame
Proportion of subjects with MLYMT scores	Proportion of subjects with MLYMT scores of 2 or more light level improvement at week 52 using the study eye	100 weeks
Proportion of subjects with MLSDT scores	Proportion of subjects with multiluminance shape discrimination test (MLSDT) scores of 2 or more light level improvements at week 52 using the study eye	100 weeks
Change from baseline in MLYMT score	Change from baseline in the MLYMT score at week 52 when using both eyes	100 weeks
Change from baseline in MLYMT score	Change from baseline in MLYMT at weeks 16, 24, 36, 52, 76, and 100	100 weeks
Proportion of MLYMT responders to treatment	Proportion of MLYMT responders to treatment at weeks 16, 24, 36, 52, 76, and 100	100 weeks
Effect of MCO-010 as assessed by static shape recognition assay	Change from baseline in accuracy in determination of three-dimensional shapes using the MLSDT at weeks 16, 24, 36, 52, 76, and 100	100 weeks
Proportion of MLSDT responders to treatment	Proportion of MLSDT responders to treatment at weeks 16, 24, 36, 52, 76, and 100	100 weeks
Effect of MCO-010 as assessed by Freiburg Visual Acuity	Change from baseline in Freiburg Visual Acuity (quantitative LogMAR score) at weeks 16, 24, 36, 52, 76, and 100	100 weeks
To evaluate the effect of MCO-010 on visual field	Change from baseline in Visual Fields measured by Humphrey 30–2 perimetry at weeks 16, 36, 52, 76, and 100	100 weeks

Other outcome measures

Outcome measure	Measure description	Time frame
Proportion of subjects demonstrating a ≥2 unit in either MLYMT or MLSDT score	Proportion of subjects demonstrating a ≥2 unit improvement from baseline in EITHER the MLYMT OR the MLSDT score at week 52 in the study eye	100 weeks
To evaluate the effect of MCO-010 on the listed safety endpoints	Incidences, nature, and severity of ocular and nonocular treatment emergent adverse events (TEAEs), Serious Adverse Events (SAEs); intraocular inflammation graded through ocular exam; intraocular pressure and retinal thickness	100 weeks

Sponsor
Nanoscope Therapeutics Inc.

Collaborators
No information provided

Investigators
- Study Chair: Dr. Samarendra Mohanty, Nanoscope Therapeutics Inc.

General Publications
No publications available.

Part IV
Other Treatments

Chapter 15
Completed Studies

United States

Study of Oral Minocycline in Treating Bilateral Cystoid Macular Edema Associated with Retinitis Pigmentosa

ClinicalTrials.gov ID NCT02140164

Sponsor National Eye Institute (NEI)
Information provided by the National Eye Institute (NEI) (Responsible Party)
Last update posted on 2017-12-05

Study Overview

Brief Summary
Background

- Some people with retinitis pigmentosa (RP) have macular edema (swelling) in the central retina. This can cause decreased central vision. The cause of macular edema is unknown, but may involve inflammation. The drug minocycline might help prevent inflammation and therefore might help treat macular edema and improve central visual function.

Objectives

- To see if minocycline helps people with RP and macular edema.

Eligibility

- People 12 years and older with RP who have macular edema in at least on eye.

J. N. Weiss, *Clinical Trials in Retinitis Pigmentosa Treatment*,
https://doi.org/10.1007/978-3-031-58799-3_15

Design

- Participants will be screened with medical and eye disease history. They will have an eye exam and blood tests. One eye with macular edema will be the study eye. If both eyes are affected, one will be designated the study eye.
- Participants will visit the clinic at least nine times over at least 14 months. The first three study visits will be monthly, then every 2 months.
- Participants will start taking minocycline after visit 3. They will take one pill twice daily for at least 1 year.
- Participants will keep a medicine diary and bring it to each visit with their pill bottle and unused pills.

At each study visit, participants will have some or all of the following tests:

- Eye and thyroid exams
- Blood and pregnancy tests
- Microperimetry: participants will press a button when they see a light on a computer screen
- Visual field measurement: participants will look at spots on a white screen to test side vision
- Electroretinogram: A person will be dark adapted by sitting in the dark for 30 min. After the placement of numbing eye drops, special contact lenses will be placed . The participant will watch flashing lights and recordings will be made.

Objective

Retinitis pigmentosa (RP) is a broad category of genetically heterogeneous diseases involving progressive visual loss by a constriction of visual field and loss of night vision. In up to one-third of patients, the peripheral vision loss can be compounded by central visual acuity loss from the development of cystic macular changes. While RP is a genetic disease, the etiology of progressive cell death, including that of associated cystoid macular edema (CME), is not completely understood. Inflammatory processes involving the activation of resident immune cells of the retina called microglia have been hypothesized to contribute. Minocycline inhibits the activation of microglia, decreasing the production of inflammatory factors implicated in RP progression. The objective of this study is to investigate the safety and possible efficacy of oral minocycline in participants with CME and RP.

Study Population

Five participants, ages 12 and older, with unilateral or bilateral CME associated with RP will be enrolled initially. However, up to an additional five participants may be enrolled to replace participants who may withdraw from the study prior to reaching the month 6 visit.

Design

This is a pilot, single-center, uncontrolled, open-label, prospective, Phase 1/2 clinical trial to evaluate minocycline as a potential treatment for CME secondary to RP. A pretreatment phase lasting two months will be instituted prior to investigational product (IP) initiation to assess the anatomical variability of CME as well as variability of other measurable parameters as part of the natural history of the disease. Participants will receive an oral dose of 100 mg (or appropriate weight adjusted pediatric dose) of minocycline twice daily for 12 months. There will be a common termination date, which will take place when the last recruited participant has received 12 months of IP. Participants who were recruited in the earlier part of the study will continue taking IP and be followed every two months until the common termination date. At each visit, participants will have visual acuity measured and will undergo optical coherence tomography (OCT) testing to measure retinal thickness. Measures of central visual field sensitivity full-field electroretinograms (ERG) and microperimetry (MP-1) will also be collected.

Outcome Measures

The primary outcome is the change in CME based on OCT measurements in the study eye at 6 months compared to pretreatment values. Secondary outcomes include changes in OCT thickness, changes in amplitude of photopic and scotopic responses on ERG testing, changes in microperimetry, and changes in visual field as measured by HVF 30–2 visual field testing at 6 months and 12 months compared to pretreatment values, as well as CME changes on OCT at 12 months compared to pretreatment values. Pretreatment measurements will be analyzed to measure the natural variability of the CME as well as to measure the variability of the functional testing. Safety outcomes will include the number and severity of adverse events (AEs). Ocular safety outcomes will be indicated by changes in visual acuity, ocular surface changes, intraocular inflammation and any other ocular changes not consistent with the natural progression of RP.

Official Title

Pilot Study to Evaluate Oral Minocycline in the Treatment of Cystoid Macular Edema Associated with Retinitis Pigmentosa

Conditions

Retinitis pigmentosa

Study Type

Interventional

Enrollment (Actual)

7

Intervention/Treatment

Drug: Minocycline

Phase

Phase1 Phase 2

Other Study ID Numbers

140,108

14-EI-0108 (Other Identifier) (OTHER: NIH Combined NeuroScience Institutional Review Board)

Study Start
2014–05

Primary Completion (Actual)
2015–11

Study Completion (Actual)
2016–06

United States
Maryland Locations

Bethesda, Maryland, United States, 20892
National Institutes of Health Clinical Center, 9000 Rockville Pike

Eligibility Criteria

Ages Eligible for Study
12 years and older (Child, Adult, Older Adult)

Accepts Healthy Volunteer
No

Sexes Eligible for Study
All

Description
Inclusion Criteria

- To be eligible, the following inclusion criteria must be met, where applicable.
- Participant must be 12 years of age or older.
- Participant (or legal guardian) must understand and sign the protocol's informed consent document.
- Participant must have evidence of retinitis pigmentosa (RP) as defined by characteristic electroretinogram (ERG) responses and visual fields.
- Participant must be able to swallow pills.
- Participant must have normal renal function and liver function or have mild abnormalities not above grade 1 as defined by the Common Terminology Criteria for Adverse Events v4.0 (CTCAE).
- Participant must agree to minimize exposure to sunlight or artificial ultraviolet (UV) rays and to wear protective clothing, sunglasses and sunscreen [minimum sun protection factor (SPF) 15] if s/he must be out in the sun.
- Any female participant of childbearing potential must have a negative pregnancy test at screening and be willing to undergo pregnancy tests throughout the study.
- Any female participant of childbearing potential and any male participant able to father children must have (or have a partner who has) had a hysterectomy or vasectomy, be completely abstinent from intercourse or must agree to practice two acceptable methods of contraception throughout the course of the study and for at least one week after investigational product (IP) discontinuation. Acceptable methods of contraception include:

- Hormonal contraception (i.e., birth control pills, injected hormones, dermal patch or vaginal ring)
- Intrauterine device
- Barrier methods (diaphragm, condom) with spermicide
- Surgical sterilization (hysterectomy or tubal ligation)

Exclusion Criteria

- A participant is not eligible if any of the following exclusion criteria are present.
  - Participant is actively receiving study therapy in another investigational study.
  - Participant is started on (or changed dosage of) topical or systemic carbonic anhydrase inhibitor (CAI) treatment in the 3 months prior to enrollment.
  - Participant is actively receiving systemic steroids or has received systemic steroids in the 3 months prior to enrollment.
  - Any female participant of childbearing potential that is pregnant, breastfeeding or planning to become pregnant during the study.
  - Participant is expected to be unable to comply with study procedures or follow-up visits.
  - Participant has evidence of an ocular disease other than RP in either eye that may confound the outcome of the study (e.g., diabetic retinopathy with 10 or more hemorrhages or microaneurysms, uveitis, pseudovitelliform macular degeneration, severe myopia).
  - Participant is on ocular or systemic medications known to be toxic to the lens, retina or optic nerve (e.g., ethambutol, chloroquine, or hydroxychloroquine).
  - Participant has a condition that would preclude participation in the study (e.g., unstable medical status including blood pressure and glycemic control) by interfering with the participant s ability to engage in the required protocol evaluation and testing and/or comply with study visits.
  - Participant has a history of chronic renal failure requiring dialysis or kidney transplant.
  - Participant has a history of chronic hepatitis or liver failure.
  - Participant has a history of thyroid cancer.
  - Participant has an allergy or hypersensitivity to minocycline or any drug in the tetracycline family.
  - Participant is currently taking a tetracycline medication.
  - Participant is taking any medication that could adversely interact with minocycline such as methoxyflurane.
  - Participant has a prior history of idiopathic intracranial hypertension.

Design Details

Primary Purpose: Treatment
Allocation: N/A
Interventional Model: Single Group Assignment
Masking: None (Open Label)

Arms and interventions

Participant group/arm	Intervention/treatment
Experimental: Minocycline Oral administration of minocycline	Drug: Minocycline • Oral dose of 100 mg (or appropriate weight-adjusted pediatric dose) of minocycline twice daily for 12 months • Other Names: – Dynacin; serial number 73419626 – Minocin; serial number 72309825 – Minocin PAC – Myrac; serial number 76589055 – Solodyn; serial number 78883462 – Vectrin; serial number 78188505

Primary outcome measures

Outcome measure	Measure description	Time frame
Change in cystoid macular edema (CME) based on optical coherence tomography (OCT) Measurements in the study eye at 6 months compared to the average of the pretreatment values	Three visits (two pretreatment and one baseline) were conducted prior to the receipt of investigational product (IP) and an average of the OCT measurements at these three visits was used as the pretreatment value	Pretreatment and 6 months

Secondary outcome measures

Outcome measure	Measure description	Time frame
Change in cystoid macular edema (CME) based on optical coherence tomography (OCT) Measurements in the study eye at 12 months compared to the average of the pretreatment values	Three visits (two pretreatment and one baseline) were conducted prior to the receipt of investigational product (IP) and an average of the OCT measurements at these three visits was used as the pretreatment value	Pretreatment and 12 months
Changes in amplitude of photopic and scotopic responses on electroretinogram (ERG) testing at 6 months as compared to the average of pretreatment values	This outcome measure will not be reported	Pretreatment and 6 months
Changes in amplitude of photopic and scotopic responses on electroretinogram (ERG) testing at 12 months as compared to the average of pretreatment values	This outcome measure will not be reported	Pretreatment and 12 months
Change in microperimetry at 6 months as compared to the average of pretreatment values	Three visits (two pretreatment and one baseline) were conducted prior to the receipt of investigational product (IP) and an average of the microperimetry measurements at these three visits was used as the pretreatment value	Pretreatment and 6 months

Change in microperimetry at 12 months as compared to the average of pretreatment values	Three visits (two pretreatment and one baseline) were conducted prior to the receipt of investigational product (IP) and an average of the microperimetry measurements at these three visits was used as the pretreatment value	Pretreatment and 12 months
change in visual field as measured by HVF 30–2 visual field testing at 6 months as compared to the average of pretreatment values	Three visits (two pretreatment and one baseline) were conducted prior to the receipt of investigational product (IP) and an average of the HVF 30–2 measurements at these three visits was used as the pretreatment value	Pretreatment and 6 months
Change in visual field as measured by HVF 30–2 visual field testing at 12 months as compared to the average of pretreatment values	Three visits (two pretreatment and one baseline) were conducted prior to the receipt of investigational product (IP) and an average of the HVF 30–2 measurements at these three visits was used as the pretreatment value	Pretreatment and 12 months
Number of study eyes achieving a 15-letter or more worsening in electronic visual acuity (EVA) at 12 months as compared to baseline	Visual Acuity was measured by a certified tester using an electronic visual acuity testing machine based on the Early Treatment Diabetic Retinopathy Study (ETDRS) method	Baseline and 12 months
Number of ocular adverse events		Study duration, up to 16 months
Number of nonocular adverse events		Study duration, up to 16 months
Number of severe adverse events		Study duration, up to 16 months

Sponsor
National Eye Institute (NEI)

Collaborators
- The Emmes Company, LLC

Investigators
- Principal Investigator: Catherine A Cukras, M.D., National Eye Institute (NEI)

General Publications

- Boughman JA, Conneally PM, Nance WE. Population genetic studies of retinitis pigmentosa. Am J Hum Genet. 1980 Mar;32(2):223–35.
- Li ZY, Possin DE, Milam AH. Histopathology of bone spicule pigmentation in retinitis pigmentosa. Ophthalmology. 1995 May;102(5):805–16. https://doi.org/10.1016/s0161-6420(95)30953-0.
- Chang GQ, Hao Y, Wong F. Apoptosis: final common pathway of photoreceptor death in rd, rds, and rhodopsin mutant mice. Neuron. 1993 Oct;11(4):595–605. https://doi.org/10.1016/0896-6273(93)90072-y.

United States/Canada/France

Study to Evaluate Safety and Tolerability of QR-421a in Subjects with RP due to Mutations in Exon 13 of the USH2A Gene (Stellar)

ClinicalTrials.gov ID NCT03780257

Sponsor ProQR Therapeutics
Information provided by ProQR Therapeutics (Responsible Party)
Last update posted on 2022-04-20

Study Overview

Brief Summary
The purpose of this study is to evaluate the safety and tolerability of QR-421a administered via intravitreal injection (IVT) in subjects with retinitis pigmentosa (RP) due to mutations in exon 13 of the USH2A gene.

Detailed Description
The purpose of this study is to evaluate the safety and tolerability of QR-421a administered via IVT in subjects with RP due to mutations in exon 13 of the USH2A gene. Subjects will receive one single IVT injection of QR-421a or sham-procedure in one eye (subject's worse eye) and will be followed up for 24 months.

Three dose levels of QR-421a will be evaluated: 50, 100, and 200 μg. Additional dose levels (e.g., 25 or 400 μg) may be evaluated based on ongoing safety and efficacy data monitoring.

Initial dose cohorts will include subjects randomized to sham-procedure or treatment with QR-421a. Additional subjects may be allocated to treatment with QR-421a in subsequent or initial dose cohorts.

Official Title
A First-in-Human Study to Evaluate the Safety and Tolerability of QR-421a in Subjects with Retinitis Pigmentosa (RP) due to Mutations in Exon 13 of the USH2A Gene.

Conditions
Retinitis Pigmentosa
Usher Syndrome Type 2
Deaf Blind
Retinal Disease
Eye Diseases
Eye Diseases, Hereditary
Eye Disorders Congenital
Vision Disorders

Study Type
Interventional

Enrollment (Actual)
20

Intervention/Treatment
Drug: QR-421a
Other: Sham-procedure (dose cohort 1&2 only)

Phase
Phase 1 Phase 2

Other Study ID Numbers
PQ-421a-001
2018–002433-38 (EudraCT Number)

Study Start (Actual)
2019-03-06

Primary Completion (Actual)
2021-10-14

Study Completion (Actual)
2021-10-14

United States
Massachusetts Locations

Boston, Massachusetts, United States, 02114
Center for Clinical Research Operations, Massachusetts Eye and Ear

Michigan Locations

Ann Arbor, Michigan, United States, 48105
University of Michigan, Kellogg Eye Center

Oregon Locations

Portland, Oregon, United States, 97239
Casey Eye Institute, Oregon Health & Science University

Texas Locations

Dallas, Texas, United States, 75231
Retina Foundation of the Southwest

Canada

Montréal, Canada, H4A 3J1
Centre for Innovative Medicine, Department of Paediatric Surgery, Montreal Children's Hospital at the McGill University Health Centre

France

Montpellier, France, 34295
Hôpital Gui de Chauliac—CHRU de Montpellier—Maladies Sensorielles Génétique

Paris, France, 75012
Centre de maladies rares CHNO des Quinze Vingts

Eligibility Criteria
Ages Eligible for Study
18 years and older (Adult, Older Adult)

Accepts Healthy Volunteer
No

Sexes Eligible for Study
All

Description

Inclusion Criteria
- Male or female, ≥ 18 years of age.
- Clinical presentation consistent with RP with Usher syndrome type 2 or nonsyndromic RP (NSRP), based on ophthalmic, audiologic, and vestibular examinations.
- A molecular diagnosis of homozygosity or compound heterozygosity for 1 or more pathogenic exon 13 mutations in the USH2A gene, based on genetic analysis upon Sponsor approval.
- Impairment of VF in the opinion of the Investigator, as determined by perimetry, with a continuous area of central field greater than or equal to 10 degrees diameter in any axis in the treatment eye, and evidence of functioning rods.
- Willing and able to comply with the protocol, follow study instructions, attend study visits as required and complete all study assessments.
- Willing and able to provide informed consent for participation prior to performing any study related procedures, and suitable verbal, auditory, written and/or tactile sign language communication as to allow informed consent to be obtained, in the opinion of the Investigator.
- No limitations to SD-OCT image collection that would prevent high quality, reliable images from being obtained in both eyes as determined by the investigator.
- Reliable perimetry measurements in both eyes, as described in the Imaging Manual and determined by the Investigator.
- Clear ocular media and adequate pupillary dilation to permit good quality retinal imaging, as assessed by the Investigator.

Exclusion Criteria
- Presence of additional nonexon 13 USH2A pathogenic mutation(s) on the USH2A allele carrying the exon 13 mutation in subjects who are compound heterozygous for mutations in exon 13.
- Presence of nonexon 13 USH2A pathogenic mutation(s) on both USH2A alleles in subjects who are homozygous for mutations in exon 13.

- Presence of pathogenic mutations in genes (other than the USH2A gene) associated with Usher syndrome Type 2 or NSRP, or other inherited retinal degenerative diseases or syndromes.
- Presence of any significant ocular or nonocular disease/disorder (or medication and/or laboratory test abnormalities) which, in the opinion of the Investigator and with concurrence of the Medical Monitor, may either put the subject at risk because of participation in the study, may influence the results of the study, or the subject's ability to participate in the study. This includes but is not limited to a subject who (1) is not an appropriate candidate for antisense oligonucleotide treatment and (2) has cystoid macular edema (CME) in the treatment eye. CME is permissible if stable for 3 months (with or without treatment). Past CME is permissible if resolved for more than 1 month.
- History or presence of ocular herpetic diseases (including herpes simplex virus, varicella zoster or cytomegalovirus) in either eye.
- Presence of any active ocular infection in either eye.
- Presence of any of the following lens opacities in the treatment eye: cortical opacity $\geq$ +2, posterior subcapsular opacity $\geq$ +2, or a nuclear sclerosis $\geq$ +2, and which are (1) clinically significant in the opinion of the Investigator and (2) would adequately prevent clinical and photographic evaluation of the retina.
- History of amblyopia in the treatment eye.
- Worse than six diopters myopia in the treatment eye.
- Receipt within 3 months prior to Screening of any intraocular or periocular surgery (including refractive surgery), or an IVT injection or planned intraocular surgery or procedure during the course of the study.
- Current treatment or treatment within the past 12 months with therapies known to influence the immune system (including but not limited to steroid implants, cytostatics, interferons, tumor necrosis factor (TNF)-binding proteins, drugs acting on immunophilins, or antibodies with known impact on the immune system). Subjects that have been treated with systemic steroids within the past 12 months or that require intermittent use of topical steroids may be considered for inclusion following approval by the Medical Monitor.
- A history of glaucoma or an IOP greater than 24 mmHg in either eye that is not controlled with medication or surgery at the time of informed consent.
- Use of any investigational drug or device within 90 days or 5 half-lives preceding the first dose of study medication, whichever is longer, or plans to participate in another study of an investigational drug or device during the PQ-421a-001 study period.
- Any prior treatment with genetic or stem-cell therapy for ocular or nonocular disease.
- History of malignancy within 5 years prior to Screening, except adequately treated squamous or basal cell carcinoma of the skin or carcinoma in situ of the cervix that has been successfully treated.
- Known hypersensitivity to antisense oligonucleotides or any constituents of the injection.
- Pregnant and breastfeeding subjects. Females of childbearing potential and males must comply with using highly effective methods of contraception as defined in Section 6.2.2. Women of nonchildbearing potential may be included without the use of adequate birth control, provided they meet the criteria in the protocol.

Design Details
Primary Purpose: Treatment
Allocation: Randomized
Interventional Model: Sequential Assignment
Masking: Quadruple (Participant Care Provider Investigator Outcomes Assessor)

Arms and interventions

Participant group/arm	Intervention/treatment
Experimental: QR-421a Single dose administration	Drug: QR-421a • RNA antisense oligonucleotide for intravitreal injection • Other Names: – RNA antisense oligonucleotide for intravitreal injection
Sham Comparator: Sham-procedure (dose cohort 1&2 only) Sham-procedure (no experimental drug administered)	Other: Sham-procedure (dose cohort 1&2 only) • Sham-procedure (no experimental drug administered) • Other Names: – Sham-procedure

Primary outcome measures

Outcome measure	Measure description	Time frame
Incidence and severity of ocular adverse events (AEs) in the treatment and contralateral eye	Incidence and severity of ocular AEs	24 months
Incidence and severity of nonocular AEs	Incidence and severity of nonocular AEs	24 months

Secondary outcome measures

Outcome measure	Measure description	Time frame
Change in DAC perimetry	Change in Dark Adapted Chromatic (DAC) perimetry	24 months
Change in static perimetry	Change in static perimetry	24 months
Change in EZ area by SD-OCT	Change in Ellipsoid Zone (EZ) area/width by spectral domain optical coherence tomography (SD-OCT)	24 months
Change in BCVA	Change in Best Corrected Visual Acuity (BCVA)	24 months
Change in LLVA	Change in Low Luminance Visual Acuity (LLVA)	24 months
Change in microperimetry	Change in microperimetry	24 months
Changes in FST	Changes in Full-field Stimulus Threshold (FST)	24 months
Changes in FAF	Changes in Fundus autofluorescence (FAF)	24 months
AUC (0-∞) of QR-421a in serum	Area under the curve 0 hour to infinity [AUC(0-∞)] of QR-421a in serum	24 months
AUC (0-tlast) of QR-421a in serum	Area under the curve 0 hour to the final sample with a concentration greater than lower limit of quantification (LLOQ) [AUC(0-tlast)] of QR-421a in serum	24 months

Cmax of QR-421a in serum	Maximum concentration (Cmax) of QR-421a in serum	24 months
Tmax of QR-421a	Time to maximum concentration (Tmax) of QR-421a	24 months
T1/2 of QR-421a	Terminal elimination half-life (T1/2) of QR-421a	24 months
Serum clearance (CL) of QR-421a	Serum clearance (CL) of QR-421a	24 months
Volume of distribution (Vd) of QR-421a	Volume of distribution (Vd) of QR-421a	24 months

Sponsor
ProQR Therapeutics

Collaborators
No information provided

Investigators
- Study Director: ProQR Medical Monitor, ProQR Therapeutics
- Study Director: ProQR Clinical Trial Manager, ProQR Therapeutics

General Publications
No publications available.

China

Cone Rescue in Retinitis Pigmentosa by the Treatment of Lycium Barbarum

ClinicalTrials.gov ID NCT02244996

Sponsor The Hong Kong Polytechnic University
Information provided by Henry HL Chan, PhD, The Hong Kong Polytechnic University (Responsible Party)
Last Update Posted 2019-02-19

Brief Summary
Objectives: To study the immediate effect and the persistent effect of Lycium barbarum (LB) treatment on retinal functions, especially the cone function, and retinal structure in patients with retinitis pigmentosa (RP) Design: Randomised controlled double-masked trial

Setting: Primary Care clinical trial

Participants: 120 RP subjects will be recruited from Ophthalmology department at the University of Hong Kong and the Retina Hong Kong. Interventions: Subjects will be randomly allocated to LB (treated with LB granules) or control (treated with placebo) groups for 1 year. After the first year, both groups will stop the treatment and all subjects will also have the same eye exam in 6-month period for the second year.

Main outcome measures: The primary outcome is the total sensitivity scores of 30–2 & 60–4 programs of Humphrey visual field analysis (HVFA). The secondary outcomes are the b-wave amplitudes of full-field electroretinogram (ffERG) responses, the amplitudes of direct component and induced component of multifocal electroretinogram (mfERG), and the ETDRS visual acuity.

Detailed Description
The study was a randomized controlled trial with a double-masked, placebo-controlled design. All the subjects were randomly allocated into either LB (treatment) group or placebo (control) group.

All the eligible subjects had the eye examination, including VA using the Early Treatment of Diabetic Retinopathy Study (ETDRS) chart, refractions, tonometry, external and internal ocular health assessments, and fundus photodocumentation. Three additional tests were conducted to investigate the functional and structural changes in the RP patients, including Ganzfeld Electroretinogram, Humphrey visual field analyser (Zeiss, Dublin, USA) and spectral-domain optical coherent tomography (SD-OCT) (Heidelberg Engineering, USA).

Official Title
Cone Rescue in Retinitis Pigmentosa by the Treatment of Lycium barbarum.

Conditions
Retinitis Pigmentosa

Study Type
Interventional

Enrollment (Actual)
50

Intervention/Treatment
Dietary Supplement: Lycium barbarum
Dietary Supplement: Placebo

Phase
Not Applicable

Other Study ID Numbers
01121876

Study Start
2014–11

Primary Completion (Actual)
2016–04

Study Completion (Actual)
2017–11

Hong Kong

Hong Kong, Hong Kong
The Hong Kong Polytechnic University

Eligibility Criteria
Ages Eligible for Study
18 Years to 70 Years (Adult, Older Adult)

Accepts Healthy Volunteer
No

Sexes Eligible for Study
All

Inclusion Criteria
- Ocular conditions:
  - Retinitis pigmentosa
  - Best corrected VA LogMAR 0.20 or better
  - Humphrey Visual Field Analysis (HVFA) 30–2 total mean defect > or = 250 Decibel
  - Intraocular pressure (IOP) <21 mmHg
  - van Herrick ratio < or = 0.5
  - No other ocular diseases
- Dietary conditions:
  - Fruit and vegetable intake <10 servings/day
  - Spinach or kale intake < or = serving/day
  - Dietary lutein intake < or = 5.4 mg/day
  - No intake of cod liver oil or omega-3 capsules
  - Dietary Lycium barbarum intake < or = 10 fruits/week
  - Supplement intake < or = 5000 IU/day of Vit. A and < or = 30 IU/day of Vit. E
  - Alcoholic consumption < or = 3 beverages/day

Exclusion Criteria
- BMI > 40
- Intake of any anticoagulants (especially Warfarin)
- Pregnant or planning to be pregnant
- Smoking
- Other clinically significant systemic diseases, e.g., diabetes, liver disease, and heart disease

Design Details
Primary Purpose: Treatment
Allocation: Randomized
Interventional Model: Parallel Assignment
Masking: Double (Participant Investigator)

Arms and interventions

Participant group/arm	Intervention/treatment
Experimental: Lycium barbarum Daily Lycium barbarum dosage: 10 g of granules for 12 months	Dietary Supplement: Lycium barbarum • Traditional Chinese Herbs • Other Names: – Wolfberry
Placebo Comparator: Placebo Placebo	Dietary Supplement: Placebo • Placebo

Primary outcome measures

Outcome measure	Measure description	Time frame
ETDRS visual acuity (high contrast)	The high contrast visual acuity will be measured at the time point of baseline and 12 months. Visual acuity is to measure the eye's ability to resolve fine detail with full refractive error correction The change of acuity (sec of arc) between 12-month time point and baseline will be provided to show the effect of interventions The changes of the treatment group will be compared with the changes of the placebo group to illustrate the treatment effect of Lycium Barbarum	12 months

Secondary outcome measures

Outcome measure	Measure description	Time frame
Visual field sensitivity	Humphrey Visual Field Analyser will be used to measure the brightness sensitivity across the central 30 degree visual field at time point of baseline and 12 months. Visual field is to measure the size of the field of view and the sensitivity of the corresponding locations of the field of view The change of sensitivity (dB) between 12-month time point and baseline will be provide to show the effects of interventions The changes of the treatment group will be compared with the changes of the placebo group to illustrate the treatment effect of Lycium barbarum	12 months
Amplitudes of flash electroretinogram	The cone responses from electroretinogram will be measured at the time point of baseline and 12 months. The cone response is related to the activity of the cone photoreceptor under light stimulation The change of cone response b-wave amplitude (uV) between 12-month and baseline will be provided to show the effect of interventions. The b-wave amplitude is to measure the magnitude of electrical responses of cone cells in the retina The changes of the treatment group will be compared with the changes of the placebo group to illustrate the treatment effect of Lycium barbarum	12 months

Implicit times of flash electroretinogram	The cone responses from electroretinogram will be measured at the time point of baseline and 12 months. The cone response is related to the activity of the cone photoreceptor under light stimulation The change of cone response b-wave implicit time (ms) between 12-month and baseline will be provided to show the effect of interventions. The b-wave implicit time is to measure the physiological changes of cone cells in the retina The changes of the treatment group will be compared with the changes of the placebo group to illustrate the treatment effect of Lycium Barbarum	12 months

Sponsor
The Hong Kong Polytechnic University

Collaborators
- The University of Hong Kong

Investigators
- Principal Investigator: Henry HL Chan, PhD, The Hong Kong Polytechnic University

General Publications
No publications available.

Italy

Nerve Growth Factor Eye Drops Treatment in Patients with Retinitis Pigmentosa and Cystoid Macular Edema (NEMO)

ClinicalTrials.gov ID NCT02609165

Sponsor Ospedale San Raffaele
Information provided by Paolo Rama, Ospedale San Raffaele (Responsible Party)
Last update posted on 2017-09-06

Study Overview

Brief Summary
This study aims at investigating the therapeutic potential of recombinant human Nerve Growth Factor (rhNGF) eye drops treatment in patients with retinitis pigmentosa (RP) associated with cystoid macular edema (CME) in a phase II, randomized, double-masked, controlled clinical trial.

Official Title
Nerve Growth Factor Eye Drops as a Novel Treatment for Vision Loss in Patients with Retinitis Pigmentosa: From Preclinical to Clinical Phase II Trial.

Conditions
Retinitis Pigmentosa
Cystoid Macular Edema

Study Type
Interventional

Enrollment (Actual)
45

Intervention/Treatment
Drug: rhNGF 180 μg/ml eye drops solution
Drug: vehicle eye drops

Phase
Phase 2

Other Study ID Numbers
RF-2010-2318561

Study Start
2015–05

Primary Completion (Actual)
2017–02

Study Completion (Actual)
2017–02

Italy

Milan, Italy, 20132
Ospedale San Raffaele

Milan, Italy
Ospedale Sacco

Eligibility Criteria
Ages Eligible for Study
18 Years and older (Adult, Older Adult)

Accepts Healthy Volunteer
No

Sexes Eligible for Study
All

Inclusion Criteria
- Typical and atypical forms of retinitis pigmentosa (RP).
- Measurable ERG with a significant decrease in the amplitude.
- Reduction of the visual field (assessed with Humphrey field analyzer- HFA 24–2) and values of mean deviation> −3 decibel (dB).

- RP associated with CME documented by OCT (macular thickness greater than 250 uM) present for at least three months and not in treatment for at least one month
- Best corrected visual acuity (BCVA) between 20/100 (2/10 or 0.1 logMAR) and 20/25 (8/10 or 0.7 logMAR) and best corrected visual acuity for near not exceeding II character.
- Absence of other ocular confounding diseases.
- Participant must be medically able to undergo the testing and study procedures required in the flowsheet of exam procedures.

Exclusion Criteria

- Presence of diabetes-related macular edema, or macular edema associated with other causes such as choroidal neovascularization or after the eye surgery.
- Patients with diabetes mellitus.
- Patients who have performed eye surgery in the previous three months.
- Evidence of an active eye infection.
- Previous uveitis or evidence of intraocular inflammation.
- History or evidence of glaucoma or elevated intraocular pressure (IOP) greater than or equal to 21 mm Hg at baseline.
- Abnormalities of the anterior segment or media opacities that prevent the assessment of the posterior segment of the eye
- The treatment with corticosteroids (systemic, periocular or intravitreal) from at least 3 months.
- The use of any topical medication other than the study drug for the treatment of ocular pathologies.
- Presence or history of any systemic or ocular disease or condition that may significantly limit of visual acuity or visual field, hindering the effectiveness of treatment in the study or its evaluation, or could interfere with the interpretation of The study results, or may be judged by the investigator incompatible with the visit program or with the procedures in the study.
- Known hypersensitivity to study drug or drugs procedural.
- Participation in another clinical study during the same period of this study or within 90 days of the screening visit / baseline.
- History of drug use, illegal drugs or alcohol abuse or addiction.
- Women of childbearing potential are excluded from participation in the study if they meet one of the following conditions:

  - Currently pregnant.
  - Have a positive urine pregnancy test at screening/baseline.
  - They plan to become pregnant during the treatment period of the study.
  - They are breastfeeding.
  - They are not available to use highly effective measures of birth control, such as: the oral hormonal contraceptives and/or mechanical barrier methods—spermicide in conjunction with a barrier such as a condom or diaphragm or during the entire course of the study and 30 days after treatment periods provided.

Design Details

Primary Purpose: Treatment
Allocation: Randomized
Interventional Model: Parallel Assignment
Masking: Quadruple (Participant Care Provider Investigator Outcomes Assessor)

Arms and interventions

Participant group/arm	Intervention/treatment
Active Comparator: study group rhNGF 180 μg/ml eye drops solution	Drug: rhNGF 180 μg/ml eye drops solution • Eye drops • Other Names: – Recombinant human Nerve Growth Factor
Placebo Comparator: control group vehicle eye drops solution	Drug: vehicle eye drops • Placebo • Other Names: – Vehicle eye drop solution

Primary outcome measures

Outcome measure	Measure description	Time frame
Macular thickness	Assessed by ocular coherence tomography (OCT)	28 days of treatment

Secondary outcome measures

Outcome measure	Measure description	Time frame
Visual field	Mean deviation	28 days of treatment, 1 month, 6 months, and 12 months of follow-up
Macular photoreceptors thickness	Assessed by OCT	28 days of treatment, 1 month, 3 months, 6 months, and 12 months of follow-up
Macular thickness	Assessed by OCT	1 month, 3 months, 6 months, and 12 months of follow-up
Electroretinogram (ERG)	Amplitudes	28 days of treatment, 1 month, 6 months, and 12 months of follow-up
Visual acuity		28 days of treatment,1 month, 3 months, 6 months, and 12 months of follow-up
Contrast sensitivity		28 days of treatment, 1 month, 3 months, 6 months, and 12 months of follow-up
Quality of life		28 days of treatment, 1 month, 3 months, 6 months, and 12 months of follow-up
Number of cystoid macular edema relapses		through study completion, up to 12 months of follow-up
Number of drop out for inefficacy of the study treatment		Through study completion, up to 12 months of follow-up
Adverse events		Through study completion, up to 12 months of follow-up

Sponsor

Ospedale San Raffaele

Collaborators

- Dompé Farmaceutici S.p.A

Investigators

- Principal Investigator: Paolo Rama, MD, Ospedale San Raffaele. Milan

General Publications

No publications available.

Turkey

Management of Cystoid Macular Edema Secondary to Retinitis Pigmentosa Via Subliminal Micropulse Yellow Laser (SL-MPL)

ClinicalTrials.gov ID NCT04234438

Sponsor Ankara Universitesi Teknokent
Information provided by Umut Arslan, Ankara Universitesi Teknokent (Responsible Party)
Last update posted on 2020-01-23

Study Overview

Brief Summary

Purpose: To investigate the effects of subliminal micropulse yellow laser application on central macular thickness and best corrected visual acuity in cystoid macular edema secondary to retinitis pigmentosa patients.

Detailed Description

Retinitis pigmentosa (RP) is a progressive photoreceptor and retinal pigment epithelial (RPE) degeneration that begins as a night vision loss, resulting in narrowing of the visual field and legal blindness. RP is a heterogeneous genetic disorder, affecting 1/3000–8000 people worldwide. RP is the result of mutation in one of more than 260 genes. These genes are responsible for the synthesis of peptides involved in the visual cycle. These genes are also responsible for the synthesis of growth factors responsible for the conversion of glucose to adenosine triphosphate (ATP) or responsible for the removal of metabolic wastes.

The incidence of cystoid macular edema (CME) in RP has been reported as between 10%–50%. There are several hypotheses about the pathogenesis of cystoid macular edema in RP. The first hypothesis is explained by Müller cell hypertrophy and its paracrine effects. Mutations in the retinal pigment epithelium disrupt the synthesis of some growth factors. Stress caused by apoptosis in rod cells in the periphery leads to ectopic synaptogenesis of Müller cells in the central. Müller cells undergo compensatory hypertrophy and synthesize excessive growth factors. This paracrine effect provides protection of central vision. Edema in a certain level is considered to be protective to photoreceptors and should not be treated. But if edema is excessive and prolonged leads to a break in synaptic connections in the neural retina and an increase in neurodegeneration. CME also deteriorates central visual quality in patients with impaired peripheral vision. Treatment should be considered only if the edema is excessive and disrupts central vision. According to our clinical experience, when central macular thickness exceeds 500 microns, central visual quality of the patient decreases and requires treatment.

Other pathophysiological causes of CME in RP are explained by low-grade inflammation and retinal autoantibodies. In some genetic mutation types of RP, such as the X-linked RPGR gene mutation; vitritis, lipofuscin deposits and inflammation are predominant. Ciliopathy leads to inflammation and CME, which increases photoreceptor loss rate. Immediate treatment of inflammation-induced edema can slow disease progression. Inflammatory edema appears as cystoid macular edema, whereas compensatory edema due to Müller cell hypertrophy is seen as separated intraretinal cysts. Inflammatory edema responds well to carbonic anhydrase inhibitors, while compensatory edema does not.

The results of the treatment of CME in RP are controversial, as the compensatory or inflammatory distinction is not made clearly. Treatments such as grid laser photocoagulation, oral acetazolamide, topical carbonic anhydrase inhibitors, intravitreal therapy with corticosteroids or antivascular endothelial growth factor agents and pars plana vitrectomy may be effective in some cases with CME secondary to RP. Most of these treatments have either insufficient response or excessive side effects.

To our knowledge, so far, we have not found a scientific publication about the use of micropulse yellow laser for treatment cystoid macular edema secondary to retinitis pigmentosa.

Subliminal micropulse laser (SL-MPL) is a method developed to reduce the laser-induced thermal damage caused by conventional laser therapy for treatment some macular diseases. In the micropulse mode, laser is applied in short pulses, thereby reducing the thermal energy generated in the target area. The coagulation scars do not form with SL-MPL treatment. Sublethally injured RPE cells induce an up- and downregulation of various growth factors (GFs) [pigment epithelium-derived factor (PEDF), vascular endothelial growth factor (VEGF) inhibitors, VEGF inducers, permeability factors, etc.] which restores the pathologic imbalance.

The aim of this study was to investigate the effect of yellow (577 nm) SL-MPL therapy on central macular thickness (CMT) and on best corrected visual acuity (BCVA) in patients with cystoid macular edema secondary to retinitis pigmentosa.

Official Title

Management of Cystoid Macular Edema Secondary to Retinitis Pigmentosa via Subliminal Micropulse Yellow Laser.

Conditions

Retinitis pigmentosa
Cystoid macular edema

Study Type

Interventional

Enrollment (Actual)
32

Intervention/Treatment
Device: SL-MPL treatment protocol was performed with a 577 nm yellow laser (EasyRet, Quantel Medical, Cedex, France)

Phase
Not applicable

Other Study ID Numbers
20-1249-17

Study Start (Actual)
2018-01-01

Primary Completion (Actual)
2019-10-30

Study Completion (Actual)
2019-12-30

Turkey
Türkiye Locations

Ankara, Türkiye, Turkey, 06312
Ankara University Biotechnology Institute

Ankara, Türkiye, Turkey, 06312
Umut Arslan

Eligibility Criteria
Ages Eligible for Study
18 years to 70 years (Adult, Older Adult)

Accepts Healthy Volunteer
No

Sexes Eligible for Study
All

Inclusion Criteria
- Diagnosis of any phenotypic variation of RP
- Presence of separated intraretinal cysts
- Central macular thickness $\geq$ 500 μm
- Unresponsive to systemic or topical carbonic anhydrase inhibitors
- No interventional treatment for macular edema in the last 3 months

Exclusion Criteria
- Patients with signs of inflammation, such as cells in the vitreous, intraretinal white dots, septa-free edema
- Patients responding to systemic or topical carbonic anhydrase inhibitors

- Any interventional treatment has been applied for macular edema in the last 3 months
- The presence of other causes that may lead to CME such as epiretinal membrane, vitreous traction, diabetes or uveitis.

Design details

Primary Purpose: Treatment
Allocation: Nonrandomized
Interventional Model: Single Group Assignment
Interventional Model Description: Prospective open-label clinical trial, included 32 eyes of 29 patients who had cystoid macular edema secondary to retinitis pigmentosa. Patients were treated by subliminal micropulse yellow laser for one session. Central macular thickness and best corrected visual acuity changes were investigated just before the treatment and 1 year later after the one session of the treatment.
Masking: None (Open Label)

Arms and interventions

Participant group/arm	Intervention/treatment
Active Comparator: Before application 32 eyes of 29 patients who had cystoid macular edema secondary to retinitis pigmentosa before subliminal micropulse laser application	Device: SL-MPL treatment protocol was performed with a 577 nm yellow laser (EasyRet, Quantel Medical, Cedex, France) • Macular laser treatment was applied after pupil dilation and topical anesthesia. Laser application was performed with a Mainster Standard contact laser lens (Volk Optical, Mentor, OH, USA). To determine the appropriate personalized calibration value, single-spot test shot was applied under the green filter to a nonedematous area of the macula outside the temporal vascular arcade. The laser power was gradually increased until it formed a barely visible laser spot. The power of the micropulse pattern laser was set at 50% of the power needed to form a barely visible laser spot. Laser parameters used were 200 ms duration, 160 μm spot diameter, low operating cycle (5%), and zero spacing with 5 × 5 pattern shape. SL-MPL was applied to the areas where edema was detected in OCT and examination.
Active Comparator: After application 32 eyes of 29 patients who had cystoid macular edema secondary to retinitis pigmentosa after 12 months subliminal micropulse laser application	Device: SL-MPL treatment protocol was performed with a 577 nm yellow laser (EasyRet, Quantel Medical, Cedex, France) • Macular laser treatment was applied after pupil dilation and topical anesthesia. Laser application was performed with a Mainster Standard contact laser lens (Volk Optical, Mentor, OH, USA). To determine the appropriate personalized calibration value, single-spot test shot was applied under the green filter to a nonedematous area of the macula outside the temporal vascular arcade. The laser power was gradually increased until it formed a barely visible laser spot. The power of the micropulse pattern laser was set at 50% of the power needed to form a barely visible laser spot. Laser parameters used were 200 ms duration, 160 μm spot diameter, low operating cycle (5%), and zero spacing with 5 × 5 pattern shape. SL-MPL was applied to the areas where edema was detected in OCT and examination

Primary outcome measures

Outcome measure	Measure description	Time frame
Central macular thickness	It is obtained by measuring the distance between the internal limiting membrane and the Bruch membrane in the center of fovea by OCT	Change from baseline central macular thickness at 12 months

Sponsor
Ankara Universitesi Teknokent

Collaborators
No information provided

Investigators
- Principal Investigator: Umut Arslan, MD, Ankara Universitesi Teknokent

General Publications
No publications available.

Chapter 16
Active, Recruiting Studies

United States

Oral Hydroxychloroquine (HCQ) for Retinitis Pigmentosa Caused by P23H-Rhodopsin (RHO)

ClinicalTrials.gov ID NCT04120883

Sponsor University of Michigan
Information provided by David Zacks, University of Michigan (Responsible Party)
Last Update Posted 2023-02-09

Brief Summary
This research study is being done to learn what effect 12 months of treatment with oral hydroxychloroquine (HCQ) will have on the retina in people with retinitis pigmentosa (RP). The hypothesis is that treatment with HCQ is safe and tolerable in patients with autosomal dominant retinitis pigmentosa (adRP) caused by P23H-RHO, and may arrest progression of retinal degeneration by altering the autophagy pathway in photoreceptors.

Participants that meet eligibility and agree to the study will be asked to take the study medication (HCQ) for 12 months and have evaluations for up to approximately 18 months from the baseline visit. There will be a total of six visits (1 is a phone visit) and will include general examinations, blood work, electrocardiograms, along with special testing of the retina.

Official Title
Oral Hydroxychloroquine for Retinitis Pigmentosa Caused by P23H-RHO (Substitution of Proline to Histidine at Codon 23 of the Rhodopsin Protein).

Conditions
Retinitis pigmentosa

J. N. Weiss, *Clinical Trials in Retinitis Pigmentosa Treatment*,
https://doi.org/10.1007/978-3-031-58799-3_16

Study Type
Interventional

Enrollment (Estimated)
12

Intervention/Treatment
Drug: Hydroxychloroquine lower dose
Drug: Hydroxychloroquine higher dose

Phase
Phase 1 Phase 2

Other Study ID Numbers
HUM00164470

Study Start (Actual)
2020-02-25

Primary Completion (Estimated)
2025-10

Study Completion (Estimated)
2025-10

Study Contact
Name: Callie Gordon
Phone number: 734-615-8560
Email: callieg@umich.edu

Study Contact Backup
Name: Yu Cheng MD Zhao, MD
Phone Number: 734-232-8262
United States
Michigan Locations

Ann Arbor, Michigan, United States, 48109
Recruiting
University of Michigan

Contact
Callie Gordon
734-615-8560 callieg@umich.edu

Eligibility Criteria
Ages Eligible for Study
18 Years and older (Adult, Older Adult)

Accepts Healthy Volunteer
No

Sexes Eligible for Study
All

Inclusion Criteria

- Stated willingness to comply with all study procedures and availability for the duration of the study
- Signed and dated informed consent form
- Early Treatment Diabetic Retinopathy Study Best Corrected Visual Acuity (ETDRS BCVA) of 20 letters (approximately 20/400 Snellen) or better in at least one eye
- Clinical diagnosis of autosomal dominant retinitis pigmentosa
- Confirmed to have one copy of the P23H-RHO pathogenic variant by genetic testing at a Clinical Laboratory Improvement Amendments (CLIA)-certified laboratory
- Clarity of ocular media and adequate pupillary dilation to allow for adequate clinical ocular examination and retinal imaging
- Ability to perform testing required by the study as determined by the investigator
- Ability to take oral medication (medication tablets must be swallowed whole) and be willing to adhere to the daily medication regimen
- For females of reproductive potential, use of highly effective contraception beginning no later than 1 week after the first screening visit, and agreement to use such a method during study participation and through the end of the washout period (6 months after the end of HCQ administration)
- Agreement to adhere to lifestyle considerations throughout study duration (take the study drug with meals, avoid taking over-the-counter antacids or kaolin-containing products 4 hours before or after taking the study drug)

Exclusion Criteria

- Use of any other drugs which are known to prolong the QT interval
- Concurrent use of any of the following drugs, if the drug cannot be discontinued or substituted: digoxin, antiepileptic medications, cimetidine, methotrexate, cyclosporine, praziquantel, and ampicillin
- Current or previous use of tamoxifen
- Pregnancy or lactation
- Known allergy or hypersensitivity to hydroxychloroquine or any other 4-aminoquinoline drugs (chloroquine, amodiaquine, mefloquine, quinacrine, etc.), or known history of glucose-6-phosphate dehydrogenase deficiency
- Treatment with another investigational medical intervention for retinitis pigmentosa within 3 months, or any previous treatment with an investigational surgical intervention
- Any preexisting cardiac, renal, hepatic, or hematologic disease, any prior history of psoriasis or porphyria, or any alcoholism
- Abnormal screening laboratory values including aspartate transaminase (AST) or alanine transaminase (ALT) >2.0 × upper limit of normal, subnormal glomerular filtration rate (<90 mL/min/1.73 m^2) or abnormal complete blood count attributable to underlying hematologic disease such as malignancy, aplastic anemia, agranulocytosis, leukopenia, or thrombocytopenia.

Design Details

Primary purpose: Treatment

Allocation: Nonrandomized

Interventional model: Sequential Assignment

Interventional model description: The start of intervention for treatment arm 2 of the study will be delayed until preliminary safety of the drug is established with the 6 patients in treatment arm 1 at the first follow-up visit (4 months).

Masking: Single (outcomes assessor)

Arms and interventions

Participant group/arm	Intervention/treatment
Experimental: HCQ treatment 1 In treatment arm 1, the dose of study drug will be 4 mg/kg/day. The daily dose will not exceed 400 mg. In both groups, the dose will be rounded down to 100, 200, 300, or 400 mg/day	Drug: Hydroxychloroquine lower dose • The participants weight will be measured and converted to kilograms. The participants will receive 4 mg/kg/day. At the first follow-up visit (4 months) weight will be remeasured and the study drug dosing will be adjusted accordingly if the dosing has changed. Participants receiving 100 mg daily will be instructed to ingest one 200 mg tablet every other day. Participants receiving 200 mg daily will be instructed to ingest one 200 mg tablet daily. Participants receiving 300 mg daily will be instructed to alternate days ingesting two 200 mg tablets and one 200 mg tablet. Participants receiving 400 mg daily will be instructed to ingest two 200 mg tablets daily • Other names – Plaquenil
Experimental: HCQ treatment 2 In treatment arm 2, the dose of the study drug will be 5 mg/kg/day. The daily dose will not exceed 400 mg. In both groups, the dose will be rounded down to 100, 200, 300, or 400 mg/day	Drug: Hydroxychloroquine higher dose • The start of intervention for treatment arm 2 of the study will be delayed until preliminary safety of the drug is established with the 6 patients in treatment arm 1 at the first follow-up visit (4 months) The participants in this group will receive 5 mg/kg/day. At the first follow-up visit (4 months) weight will be remeasured and the study drug dosing will be adjusted accordingly if the dosing has changed. Participants receiving 100 mg daily will be instructed to ingest one 200 mg tablet every other day. Participants receiving 200 mg daily will be instructed to ingest one 200 mg tablet daily. Participants receiving 300 mg daily will be instructed to alternate days ingesting two 200 mg tablets and one 200 mg tablet. Participants receiving 400 mg daily will be instructed to ingest two 200 mg tablets daily. • Other names: – Plaquenil

Primary outcome measures

Outcome measure	Measure description	Time frame
Change in ellipsoid zone area measured by spectral-domain optical coherence tomography (SD-OCT)	These will be performed at: screening, baseline, 4 months, 12 months, and 18 months	Screening up to 18 months
Change in retinal sensitivity (decibels) measured by scotopic and mesopic microperimetry	These will be performed at: screening, baseline, 4 months, 12 months, and 18 months	Screening up to 18 months

Sponsor
University of Michigan

Collaborators
Cures Within Reach

Investigators
Principal Investigator: David Zacks, MD, University of Michigan

General Publications
No publications available

Active, Recruiting

United States

Sildenafil for Treatment of Choroidal Ischemia

ClinicalTrials.gov ID NCT04356716

Sponsor Columbia University
Information provided by Columbia University (Responsible Party)
Last Update Posted 2022-05-06

Brief Summary
The hypothesis of this study is to determine if there is a benefit afforded by the use of systemic sildenafil to patients with choroidal and retinal degenerations and dystrophies, such as vitelliform degeneration, dry and reticular age-related macular degeneration (AMD) as well as patients with hereditary and acquired retinal dystrophies such as retinitis pigmentosa and central serous retinopathy.

Detailed Description
Age-related macular degeneration (AMD) is a sight-threatening visual disturbance that affects the macula in older ages. It is irreversible if the pigment epithelium is lost (dry AMD), but wet AMD can be arrested or delayed with the use of intraocular injections of one of the three different compounds. All the three drugs are injected into the eye in minute doses of usually 0.1 ml. These are usually injected at 4–6 week intervals and treatment may be extended for several years.

Different patterns of injection times are followed but usually are monthly for 12 or more months, or monthly for 3 months and then extended observation at one to two month intervals unless vision (visual acuity) declines or optical coherence tomography-angiography (OCT-A) shows recurrence of fluid or increase in size or amount of drusen (deposits of lipofuscin) in the retina.

Vitelliform macular degeneration is a disorder that causes visual loss due to drusen in the macula, which have been shown to be identical to the deposits seen in macular degeneration. The goal of therapy in this proposal is to use sildenafil to increase choroidal blood flow to treat dry AMD and slow the progression of visual loss in vitelliform and age-related dry AMD as well as other macular, retinal and choroidal degenerations, and dystrophies, as well as reduce or eliminate the number of injections required by slowing down transformation of dry AMD to wet AMD in treated patients.

Official Title
Sildenafil for Treatment of Choroidal Ischemia

Conditions
Choroidal ischemia
Vitelliform macular dystrophy
Age-related macular degeneration
Central serous retinopathy
Retinitis pigmentosa

Study Type
Interventional

Enrollment (Estimated)
25

Intervention/Treatment
Drug: Sildenafil
Other: Standard of care sildenafil
Diagnostic Test: Ocular coherence tomography-angiography (OCT-A)
Other: Visual acuity (VA)

Phase
Phase 2

Other Study ID Numbers
AAAM7406

Study Start (Actual)
2014-11-11

Primary Completion (Estimated)
2022-12

Study Completion (Estimated)
2022-12

Study Contact
Name: Suzanne Daly, RN, BSN
Email: sd2798@cumc.columbia.edu
United States
New York Locations

New York, New York, United States, 10032
Recruiting
Columbia University Medical Center, Edward Harkness Eye Institute

Contact
Suzanne Daly, RN, BSN
sd2798@cumc.columbia.edu

Eligibility Criteria
Ages Eligible for Study
18 Years and older (Adult, Older Adult)

Accepts Healthy Volunteer
No

Sexes Eligible for Study
All

Inclusion Criteria
- Diagnosis of retinal and choroidal degenerations (reticular or vitelliform AMD or vitelliform-type subretinal drusen) or hereditary or acquired retinal dystrophies (retinitis pigmentosa or central serous retinopathy)

Exclusion Criteria
- Diagnosis of heart disease requiring use of nitrates
- Inability to be examined monthly or bimonthly

Design Details
Primary purpose: Treatment
Allocation: Nonrandomized
Interventional model: Parallel assignment
Interventional model description: Participants are assigned to the investigational sildenafil arm with a dose of 40–80 mg daily, or the records review arm when taking sildenafil off-label.
Masking: None (open label)

Arms and interventions

Participant group/arm	Intervention/treatment
Active comparator: Standard of care sildenafil Medical record review for participants that are prescribed sildenafil off-label as part of standard of care treatment for disease.	Other: Standard of care sildenafil • Medical record review of participants that receive Sildenafil as part of standard of care • Other names: – Viagra – Revatio

Active comparator: Sildenafil Participants are prescribed sildenafil 40–80 mg daily	Drug: Sildenafil • Initial Sildenafil dosage will be weight dependent. Participants will start at 40 mg daily (20 mg in the morning, 20 mg in the evening) or 60 mg daily (40 mg in the morning and 20 mg in the evening). Sildenafil dosage may be increased to up to 80 mg daily (20–40 mg in the morning and 20–40 mg in the evening) based on the response to lower doses. If the participant has not had improvement after initial treatment, the dose may be increased, at the discretion of the study physician • Other names: – Viagra – Revatio Diagnostic test: ocular coherence tomography-angiography (OCT-A) • Retinal photographs will be taken at each study visit Other: Visual Acuity (VA) • Visual acuity will be measured with Snellen Eye chart at each study visit

Primary outcome measures

Turkey	Measure description	Time frame
Change in choroidal perfusion	Patients are evaluated for progression of disease/dystrophy via visual acuity (improved/stable/worsened) and appearance of fluid layer and drusen on OCT testing.	Up to 5 years

Sponsor
Columbia University

Collaborators
No information provided

Investigators
Principal Investigator: Donald Jackson Coleman, MD, Columbia University

General Publications

- Coleman DJ, Silverman RH, Rondeau MJ, Lloyd HO, Khanifar AA, Chan RV. Age-related macular degeneration: choroidal ischaemia? Br J Ophthalmol. 2013;97(8):1020–3. https://doi.org/10.1136/bjophthalmol-2013-303143. Epub 2013 Jun 5.
- Coleman DJ, Lee W, Chang S, Silverman RH, Lloyd HO, Daly S, Tsang SH. Treatment of Macular Degeneration with Sildenafil: Results of a Two-Year Trial. Ophthalmologica. 2018;240(1):45-54. https://doi.org/10.1159/000486105. Epub 2018 Apr 25.

Active, Recruiting

Australia

Safety and Efficacy of NPI-001 Tablets for RP Associated with Usher Syndrome (SLO RP)

ClinicalTrials.gov ID NCT04355689

Sponsor Nacuity Pharmaceuticals, Inc.
Information provided by Nacuity Pharmaceuticals, Inc. (Responsible Party)
Last Update Posted 2022-11-18

Brief Summary
This study will examine the safety and efficacy of NPI-001 Tablets as compared to placebo for 24 months in subjects with vision loss due to RP associated with Usher syndrome.

Detailed Description
This study will examine the safety and efficacy of oral NPI-001 Tablets as compared to oral placebo tablets for 24 months in subjects with vision loss due to RP associated with Usher syndrome.

Official Title
Safety and Efficacy of NPI-001 Tablets Versus Placebo for Treatment of Retinitis Pigmentosa Associated with Usher Syndrome

Conditions
Usher syndromes

Study Type
Interventional

Enrollment (Estimated)
48

Intervention/Treatment
Drug: NPI-001
Other: Placebo

Phase
Phase 1 Phase 2

Other Study ID Numbers
C-18-04
Study start (actual)
2020-09-03

Primary Completion (Estimated)
2025-01

Study Completion (Estimated)
2025-01

Study Contact
Name: Jami Kern, PhD
Phone number: +1-817-336-3000
Email: info@nacuity.com

Study Contact Backup
Name: G. Michael Wall, PhD
Phone Number: +1-817-336-3000
Email: info@nacuity.com
Australia

Brisbane, Australia
Recruiting
Queensland Eye Institute

Contact
Research Manager
Melbourne, Australia
Recruiting
CERA

Contact
Research Manager
Perth, Australia
Recruiting
Lions Eye Institute

Contact
Research Manager

Eligibility Criteria
Ages Eligible for Study
18 Years and older (Adult, Older Adult)

Accepts Healthy Volunteer
No

Sexes Eligible for Study
All

Description

Inclusion Criteria
- Male or female, age ≥18 years.
- Able to comprehend and willing to sign an informed consent form (ICF) and to adhere to the study protocol.
- Diagnosed with Usher syndrome.

- EZ zone with width ≥500 microns, which includes the fovea in each eye at Visit 2, (Screen B).
- Have at least 20 detectable points on the MAIA grid.
- On stable dose of medications associated with other conditions for at least one month.
- Both female participants of childbearing potential and male participants able to father children must have (or have a partner who has) had a bilateral oophorectomy, hysterectomy or bilateral salpingectomy; must abstain from intercourse; or must agree to practice 2 acceptable methods of contraception throughout the course of the study and 4 weeks after the last visit. Acceptable methods of contraception include hormonal contraception (i.e., birth control pills, injected hormones, dermal patch or vaginal ring), intrauterine device, barrier methods (diaphragm, condom) with spermicide, tubal ligation, or vasectomy.

Exclusion Criteria

Ocular

- All edges of the EZ area in both eyes cannot be visualized at Visit 2 (Screen B).
- Concurrent retinal pathologies that result in vision loss or inability to fixate, including but not limited to, choroideremia, retinal vein occlusion, and neovascular age-related macular degeneration.
- Intraocular surgery within the last two months or capsulotomy within the last month.
- History of uveitis, Coat's disease, diabetic retinopathy, glaucoma, herpes simplex of the eye, or currently has a cataract that prevents visualization of the posterior pole.
- Unstable fixation during microperimetry in either eye at either screening or baseline visits.

Nonocular

- Use of any other investigational new drug, or participation in another clinical trial within 12 weeks before the start of study treatment.
- Use of N-acetylcysteine containing products in the previous 30 days prior to the baseline visit or unwilling to refrain from such supplements for the duration of the study.
- Liver or kidney disease, cystic fibrosis, asthma or chronic obstructive pulmonary disease (COPD), history of thrombocytopenia not due to a reversible cause, or other blood dyscrasia.
- Suspected liver dysfunction determined by having alanine aminotransferase (ALT), aspartate aminotransferase (AST), or bilirubin values >1.5 × the upper limit of normal (ULN).
- Platelet or hemoglobin values that are below the lower limit of normal at screening (subjects with normal hemoglobin and mean corpuscular volume below the lower limit of normal should have iron studies performed to ensure that they are iron replete before taking part in the study), or neutrophils or white cell count which is above the upper limit of normal.

- Presence of more than + proteinuria on urinalysis at screening or (confirmed by abnormal albumin creatinine ratio).
- Presence of hematuria on urinalysis at screening. (If hematuria is detected on urinalysis, then the specimen should be subjected to microscopy, and subject should be excluded if more than 10×10^6 red blood cells/L). If the subject is a female in whom the hematuria may be due to menses, then the urinalysis can be repeated after a few days.
- C-reactive protein (CRP) value above 10 mg/L.
- Subject has a recent history of presence of gross blood in stools.
- History of known sensitivity to N-acetylcysteine or similar thiol compounds.
- History of hypersensitivity to any medication or food resulting in systemic symptoms.
- History of cancer (other than nonmelanoma skin cancer) diagnosed or requiring treatment within the past 2 years.
- Pregnant women or women planning to become pregnant in the next 25 months or men with partners planning to become pregnant in the next 25 months.
- Lactating women who are breastfeeding.
- A potential participant lives in the same household as a current participant in this study.
- Inability to provide blood samples, including difficulty with venous access.
- Any reason, in the opinion of the Principal Investigator, the subject should not participate.

Design Details
Primary purpose: Treatment
Allocation: Randomized
Interventional model: Parallel assignment
Interventional model description: NPI-001 Tablets versus Placebo
Masking: Quadruple (Participant Care Provider Investigator Outcomes Assessor)
Masking description: Double-masked

Arms and interventions

Participant group/arm	Intervention/treatment
Experimental: NPI-001 NPI-001 Tablet, 250 mg, BID	Drug: NPI-001 • Oral tablet
Placebo comparator: Placebo Placebo tablet, BID	Other: Placebo • Placebo tablets

Primary outcome measures

Outcome measure	Measure description	Time frame
Evaluate change from baseline for retinal sensitivity assessed by microperimetry of active versus placebo	Evaluate change from baseline for retinal sensitivity assessed by microperimetry of active versus placebo	24 months

Sponsor
Nacuity Pharmaceuticals, Inc.

Collaborators
Foundation Fighting Blindness

Investigators
Study Chair: Lee Anderson, MD, Nacuity Pharmaceuticals, Inc.

General Publications
No publications available

Active, Recruiting

China

Minocycline Treatment in Retinitis Pigmentosa

ClinicalTrials.gov ID NCT04068207

Sponsor Sun Yat-sen University
Information provided by Dan Liang, Sun Yat-sen University (Responsible Party)
Last update posted on 2023-04-18

Study Overview

Brief Summary
The aim of this study is to evaluate the efficacy and safety of oral minocycline (100 mg/day), administered for 6 months, for the treatment of patients with retinitis pigments (RP).

Detailed Description
Retinitis pigmentosa (RP) is a sort of inherited blinding disorders, and no effective or safe treatment is widely applied for it. The worldwide prevalence of RP is estimated to be 1/5000. RP is characterized by the degeneration of peripheral rod photoreceptor (PR) and associated retinal pigment epithelium (RPE) cells. Nyctalopia and visual field constriction are common symptoms. Cone degeneration and associated loss of central vision are typically followed later.

Minocycline, a second-generation, semisynthetic tetracycline antibiotic, is a highly lipophilic molecule and can easily pass through the blood-brain barrier. Several animal experiments and clinical trials have reported that minocycline exert antiapoptotic, antiinflammatory, and antioxidant effects in treating neurodegenerative diseases.

We propose to test the effect and safety of oral minocycline for retinitis pigmentosa.

Official Title
The Efficacy and Safety of Oral Minocycline in the Treatment of Retinitis Pigmentosa: An Open-label Clinical Trial

Conditions
Retinitis pigmentosa
Inherited retinal dystrophy
Retina disorder

Study Type
Interventional

Enrollment (Estimated)
35

Intervention/Treatment
Drug: Minocycline

Phase
Phase 2

Other Study ID Numbers
5010-MINO-RP

Study Start (Actual)
2019-02-22

Primary Completion (Actual)
2021-09-01

Study Completion (Estimated)
2023-12-01

Study Contact
Name: Dan Liang, MD
Phone Number: 0086-20-87330402
Email: liangd2@mail.sysu.edu.cn
China
Guangdong Locations

Guangzhou, Guangdong, China, 510060
Recruiting
Zhongshan Ophthalmic Center, Sun Yat-sen University

Contact
Dan Liang, MD
0086-20-87330402 liangd2@mail.sysu.edu.cn
Principal Investigator:
Dan Liang, MD

Guangzhou, Guangdong, China, 510060
Recruiting
Zhongshan Ophthalmic Center, Sun Yat-sen University

Contact
Dan Liang
0086-20-87330402 liangd2@mail.sysu.edu.cn
Principal Investigator:
Dan Liang, MD

Eligibility Criteria
Ages Eligible for Study
18–60 Years (Adult)

Accepts Healthy Volunteer
No

Sexes Eligible for Study
All

Description

Inclusion Criteria
- Clinical diagnosis of retinitis pigmentosa: nyctalopia, visual field constriction, and loss of central vision; degeneration of peripheral rod photoreceptor and retinal pigment epithelium cells.
- Aged from 18 to 60 years old.
- BCVA >20/100 (0.2).
- Full-field cone electroretinogram amplitude to 30-Hz flashes >0 uV.
- Written informed consent is provided.

Exclusion Criteria
- Glucocorticoids or tetracycline were used within 3 months.
- Vitamin A, DHA, and other neurotrophic drugs were used within 3 months.
- Other ocular diseases or fundus diseases except cataract: glaucoma, diabetic retinopathy, and retinal detachment.
- Tetracycline or minocycline allergy or intolerance.
- Renal or hepatic insufficiency.
- History of thyroid neoplasm.
- History of idiopathic intracranial hypertension.
- Pregnant or lactating females.

Design Details
Primary purpose: Treatment
Allocation: N/A
Interventional model: Single Group Assignment
Masking: None (open label)

Arms and interventions

Participant group/arm	Intervention/treatment
Experimental: Minocycline Tablets Minocycline 100 mg po/day for 24 weeks	Drug: Minocycline • Tab. Minocycline 100 mg po/day for 24 weeks • Other names: – Minocin – Minocyclinum – Minocyclin

Primary outcome measures

Outcome measure	Measure description	Time frame
Change of full-field cone electroretinogram amplitude to 30-Hz flashes	Increase of full-field cone electroretinogram amplitude to 30-Hz flashes	24 weeks

Secondary outcome measures

Outcome measure	Measure description	Time frame
Change of visual field area	HFA30-2 and HFA60-4	24 weeks
Best corrected visual acuity	Increase of BCVA	24 weeks
Central foveal thickness	Increase of central foveal thickness	24 weeks

Sponsor
Sun Yat-sen University

Collaborators
No information provided

Investigators
Principal Investigator: Dan Liang, MD, Zhongshan Ophthalmic Center, Sun Yat-sen University

General Publications
No publications available

Chapter 17
Active, Not Recruiting Studies

United States

FIGHT-RP 1 Extension Study

ClinicalTrials.gov ID NCT03999021

Sponsor Johns Hopkins University
Information provided by Johns Hopkins University (Responsible Party)
Last update posted on 2023-09-13

Brief Summary
Retinitis pigmentosa (RP) is a devastating eye disease, and at present, there are no known treatment options that can alter the rate of vision loss and eventual blindness. In a series of studies in animal models, the effects of exposing cones in the periphery of the retina to a large excess of oxygen result in progressive oxidative damage to cone photoreceptors and cone cell death. Cone cell death gradually spreads from the periphery of the retina toward its center, narrowing the visual field and eventually resulting in tunnel vision. Compared to control patients, those with RP showed significant reduction in the reduced to oxidized glutathione ratio (GSH/GSSG) in aqueous humor and a significant increase in protein carbonyl content. This demonstration of oxidative stress and oxidative damage in the eyes of patients with RP suggests that oxidative damage-induced cone cell death in animal models of RP may translate to humans with RP and support the hypotheses that (1) potent antioxidants will promote cone survival and function in patients with RP and (2) aqueous GSH/GSSG ratio and carbonyl content on proteins provide useful biomarkers of disease activity in this patient population. Orally administered N-acetylcysteine (NAC) has been found to be a particularly effective antioxidant that promotes prolonged cone survival and maintenance of cone function in a mouse model of RP. Since oral and/or topical administration of NAC is feasible for long-term

J. N. Weiss, *Clinical Trials in Retinitis Pigmentosa Treatment*,
https://doi.org/10.1007/978-3-031-58799-3_17

treatment in humans, and NAC has a good safety profile, there is good rationale to test the effect of NAC in patients with RP.

Oxidative damage has been implicated in several diseases including cystic fibrosis, chronic obstructive pulmonary disease (COPD), and idiopathic pulmonary fibrosis. The effect of oral NAC has been tested in these indications in several clinical trials providing extensive safety data. In COPD, NAC 600 mg bid improves airway function and reduces the frequency of acute exacerbations. Doses of up to 1800 mg/day have been well tolerated in the treatment of idiopathic pulmonary fibrosis. Paracetamol (acetaminophen) toxicity is treated with a loading dose of 140 mg/kg NAC followed by 70 mg/kg every 4 h for 17 doses. Normal volunteers tolerated a dose of 11.2 g NAC/day for 3 months without any serious undesirable effects, and in another study, a dose of 500 mg/kg/day was tolerated. The most frequent adverse events associated with the oral administration of NAC are gastrointestinal in nature and include vomiting, diarrhea, stomatitis, abdominal pain, and nausea (incidence rate >1/1000 to <1/100).

Hypersensitivity reactions including anaphylactic shock and anaphylactic/anaphylactoid reaction (incidence rate <1/10,000), dyspnea, bronchospasm (incidence rate >1/10,000 to <1/1000), angioedema, tachycardia, urticaria, rash, and pruritus (incidence rate >1/1000 to <1/100) have been reported less frequently. Finally, reports of headache, tinnitus, pyrexia, blood pressure decreased (incidence rate >1/1000 to <1/100), face edema and hemorrhage have also been collected with oral NAC.

In the FIGHT-RP 1 study, the investigators used escalating doses of NAC effervescent tablets (from 600 mg in Cohort 1 to 1800 mg in Cohort 3). The maximum tolerated dose was 1800 mg twice a day which will be continued in this study.

Official Title
A Phase 1 Open-Label Extension Study to Assess the Long-Term Safety and Tolerability of N-Acetylcysteine (NAC) in Patients with Retinitis Pigmentosa

Conditions
Retinitis Pigmentosa

Study Type
Interventional

Enrollment (Estimated)
30

Intervention/Treatment
Drug: NAC effervescent tablets

Phase
Phase 1

Other Study ID Numbers
IRB00204017

Study Start (Actual)
2019-06-24

Primary Completion (Estimated)
2025-02

Study Completion (Estimated)
2025-12

United States
Maryland Locations

Baltimore, Maryland, United States, 21287
Wilmer Eye Institute at Johns Hopkins University

Ages Eligible for Study
18 years and older (adult, older adult)

Accepts Healthy Volunteer
No

Sexes Eligible for Study
All

Description

Inclusion Criteria
- Age 18 years
- Patients diagnosed with RP

Informed Consent
- Authorization of use and disclosure of protected health information

Exclusion Criteria
- Patients with a concomitant ocular pathology that limits central macular function, including but not limited to age-related macular degeneration, diabetic retinopathy, and retinal vein occlusion
- Patients with an active ocular infection
- Patients with uncontrolled hypertension (defined as diastolic blood pressure >95 mmHg or systolic blood pressure >160 mmHg despite medical therapy)

Design Details
Primary Purpose: Treatment
Allocation: N/A
Interventional Model: Single Group Assignment
Masking: None (Open Label)

Arms and interventions

Participant group/ arm	Intervention/treatment
Experimental: Experimental arm All participants to receive study intervention	Drug: NAC effervescent tablets • After completing the pretreatment visits, all patients will enter into the treatment phase where patients will receive 1800 mg of NAC effervescent tablets twice a day. The patients will be followed up every 3 months for 2 years. Therefore, there will be a total of nine treatment visits (baseline, months 3, 6, 9, 12, 15, 18, 21, and 24)

Primary outcome measures

Outcome measure	Measure description	Time frame
Blood pressure (mmHg)	Blood pressure in mmHg will be used in assessing tolerability of N-Acetylcysteine	Up to 2 years
Tolerability of N-Acetylcysteine as assessed by drug-related symptoms	Participants will be assessed for the occurrence of any drug-related symptoms which includes nausea, stomach upset, diarrhea, heartburn, constipation, and vomiting. Based on the number and severity of the symptoms, the physician would conclude whether the patient is tolerating the medication or not	Up to 2 years
Tolerability of N-Acetylcysteine as assessed by time at which medication is taken	Medication diary provided to participants will be reviewed to see if participants are taking the medication within the designated time frame	Up to 2 years
Tolerability of N-Acetylcysteine as assessed by number of times medication is taken per day	Medication diary provided to participants will be reviewed to see if participants are taking the medication twice a day	Up to 2 years

Secondary outcome measures

Outcome measure	Measure description	Time frame
Change in best corrected visual acuity (BCVA)	Scoring is determined by the number of letters gained or lost per month using Early Treatment Diabetic Retinopathy Study (ETDRS) Letter Score and visual acuity score together with an overall score range of 0 to 20/20 where 0 is the worst vision and 20/20 is the best	Baseline, every 3 months up to 2 years
Change in central retinal sensitivity as assessed by microperimetry	Microperimetry (MAIA) is used to test whether there is an increase or decrease in sensitivity (dB) in the retina after initiation of N-Acetylcysteine	Baseline, every 3 months up to 2 years
Change in ellipsoid zone (EZ) width (μm)	This will be assessed by spectral domain optical coherence tomography (SD-OCT) after initiation of N-Acetylcysteine	Baseline, every 3 months up to 2 years
Change in aqueous reduced to oxidized glutathione ratio (GSH/GSSG)	This will be calculated from the proportions of reduced glutathione and oxidized glutathione in the aqueous	Baseline, every 3 months up to 2 years
Change in serum carbonyl content (nmol/mg)		Baseline, every 3 months up to 2 years
Change in aqueous levels of N-Acetylcysteine (mg)		Baseline, every 6 months up to 2 years
Change in plasma levels of N-Acetylcysteine (μg/ml)		Baseline, every 3 months up to 2 years

Sponsor
Johns Hopkins University

Collaborators
No information provided

Investigators
Principal Investigator: Peter Campochiaro, Johns Hopkins University

General Publications
No publications available

Active, Not Recruiting

United States

A Study to Evaluate the Safety and Tolerability of QR-1123 in Subjects With Autosomal Dominant Retinitis Pigmentosa Due to the P23H Mutation in the RHO Gene (AURORA)

ClinicalTrials.gov ID NCT04123626

Sponsor ProQR Therapeutics
Information provided by ProQR Therapeutics (Responsible Party)
Last Update Posted 2022-05-06

Study Overview

Brief Summary
This study evaluates the safety, tolerability, and efficacy of QR-1123 injection in the eye (intravitreal; IVT) injections (one eye/unilateral) in subjects receiving a single dose or repeat doses. Single injections will be assessed in an open label way, and repeat injections will be assessed in a double-masked, randomized, sham-controlled fashion.

Detailed Description
QR-1123 is an antisense oligonucleotide, designed to specifically target the mutant P23H messenger ribonucleic acid (mRNA) in order to reduce the expression of the P23H protein selectively, while preserving expression of the wild-type (WT) rhodopsin (RHO) protein. It is hypothesized that the reduction of mutant P23H mRNA will reduce the deleterious effects of the dominant-negative protein and should result in increased function of WT rhodopsin protein in photoreceptors. Restoration of WT RHO function is expected to improve vision in patients with adRP due to the P23H mutation.

The study will comprise up to eight single dose and repeat dose cohorts. Prior to initiating a higher single dose cohort and/or prior to initiating repeat dose cohort(s), available safety and efficacy data will be reviewed by the DMC.

In the single dose cohort, subjects will receive a single, unilateral IVT injection of QR-1123 in an open label fashion. In the repeat dose cohort, subjects will be randomized to receive either a unilateral IVT injection of QR-1123 every 3 months or a unilateral sham procedure every 3 months, in a double masked fashion. Subjects will be followed for safety, tolerability, and efficacy for a total period of 12 months.

Official Title

A Prospective First-In-Human Study to Evaluate the Safety and Tolerability of QR-1123 in Subjects with Autosomal Dominant Retinitis Pigmentosa (adRP) due to the P23H Mutation in the RHO Gene

Intervention/Treatment

Drug: QR-1123
Other: Sham procedure

Other Study ID Numbers

PQ-1123-001

Study Start (Actual)

2019-10-07

Primary Completion (Estimated)

2022-06-07

Study Completion (Estimated)

2022-06-07

Enrollment (Actual)

11

Study Type

Interventional

Phase

Phase 1 Phase 2

United States
Colorado Locations

Aurora, Colorado, United States, 80045
Sue Anschutz-Rogers Eye Center, University of Colorado - Dept. of Ophthalmology

Florida Locations

Gainesville, Florida, United States, 32607
Vitreo Retinal Associates

Kentucky Locations

Lexington, Kentucky, United States, 40536
Shriners UK Ophthalmology - University of Kentucky

Oregon Locations

Portland, Oregon, United States, 97239
Casey Eye Institute, OHSU

Texas Locations
Dallas, Texas, United States, 75231
Retina Foundation of the Southwest

Main Inclusion Criteria

- Male or female, $\geq$18 years of age.
- Clinical presentation consistent with adRP, based on ophthalmic examinations.
- Impairment on VF in the opinion of the Investigator, as determined by perimetry.
- A molecular diagnosis of autosomal dominant form of RP with the P23H mutation in the RHO gene, based on genetic analysis.
- A clear ocular media and adequate pupillary dilation to permit good quality fundus imaging, as assessed by the Investigator.

Main Exclusion Criteria

- Presence of additional pathogenic mutations in genes (other than the P23H mutation in the RHO gene) associated with inherited retinal degenerative diseases or syndromes, based on genetic analysis (e.g., Usher syndrome, Leber congenital amaurosis, etc.).
- Presence of any significant ocular or nonocular disease/disorder (including medication and laboratory test abnormalities) which, in the opinion of the Investigator and with concurrence of the Medical Monitor, may either put the subject at risk because of participation in the study, may influence the results of the study, or the subject's ability to participate in the study.

Ages Eligible for Study
18 Years and Older (Adult, Older Adult)

Sexes Eligible for Study
All

Accepts Healthy Volunteers
No

Design Details
Primary Purpose: Treatment
Allocation: Randomized
Interventional Model: Sequential Assignment
Masking: Triple (Participant Care Provider Outcomes Assessor)
Masking Description: Single dose cohorts are open label. Repeat dose cohorts are randomized, double masked.

Arms and interventions

Participant group/arm	Intervention/treatment
Experimental: QR-1123 single dose–dose level 1 Open label single dose cohort: dose level 1	Drug: QR-1123 • Unilateral IVT injection
Experimental: QR-1123 single dose–dose level 2 Open label single dose cohort: dose level	Drug: QR-1123 • Unilateral IVT injection
Experimental: QR-1123 single dose–dose level 3 Open label single dose cohort: dose level 3	Drug: QR-1123 • Unilateral IVT injection
Experimental: QR-1123 single dose–dose level 4 Open label single dose cohort: dose level 4	Drug: QR-1123 • Unilateral IVT injection
Experimental: QR-1123 single dose–dose level 5 Open label single dose cohort: dose level 5	Drug: QR-1123 • Unilateral IVT injection
Experimental: Repeat dose cohort 1 Double-masked, randomized, sham controlled, repeat dose cohort. Dose levels will be determined following DMC review of obtained safety and efficacy data	Drug: QR-1123 • Unilateral IVT injection Other: Sham procedure • Sham procedures (i.e., no penetration of the globe) closely mimic the active injection and serve to mask subjects to treatment assignment

Primary outcome measures

Outcome measure	Measure description	Time frame
Incidence and severity of ocular AEs	Incidence and severity of ocular adverse events scored based on CTCAC in the study and fellow eye	Up to 12 months
Incidence and severity of nonocular AEs	Incidence and severity of nonocular adverse events scored based on CTCAC in the study and fellow eye	Up to 12 months

Secondary outcome measures

Outcome measure	Measure description	Time frame
Changes in BCVA	Changes in best corrected visual acuity (BCVA)	Up to 12 months
Changes in LLVA	Changes in low-luminance visual acuity (LLVA)	Up to 12 months
Changes in DAC perimetry	Changes in dark adapted chromatic (DAC) perimetry	Up to 12 months
Changes in static VF	Changes in static VF (visual field)	Up to 12 months
Changes in microperimetry	Changes in microperimetry	Up to 12 months
Changes in SD-OCT	Changes in spectral domain-optical coherence tomography	Up to 12 months
Changes in FST	Changes in full-field stimulus threshold (FST)	Up to 12 months
Changes in full-field ERG	Changes in full-field electroretinogram (ERG)	Up to 12 months
Assessment of systemic exposure after treatment with QR-1123	Serum levels of QR-1123	Up to 12 months

Sponsor
ProQR therapeutics

Collaborators
No information provided

Investigators
Study Director: ProQR Medical Monitor, ProQR Therapeutics
Study Director: ProQR Clinical Trial Manager, ProQR Therapeutics

General Publications
No publications available

Active, Not Recruiting

United States/Europe

Study to Evaluate the Efficacy Safety and Tolerability of Ultevursen in Subjects with RP due to Mutations in Exon 13 of the USH2A Gene (Sirius)

ClinicalTrials.gov ID NCT05158296

Sponsor ProQR Therapeutics
Information provided by ProQR Therapeutics (Responsible Party)
Last Update Posted 2022-09-16

Study Overview

Brief Summary
The purpose of this study is to evaluate the efficacy safety and tolerability of ultevursen administered via intravitreal injection (IVT) in subjects with Retinitis Pigmentosa (RP) due to mutations in exon 13 of the USH2A gene.

Detailed Description
The purpose of this study is to evaluate the efficacy safety and tolerability of ultevursen administered via intravitreal injection (IVT) in subjects with Retinitis Pigmentosa (RP) due to mutations in exon 13 of the USH2A gene.

The below dose levels of ultevursen will be evaluated with the loading dose administered at Day 1 and maintenance dose administered at Month 3 and every 6 months thereafter:

1. Loading dose of 180 μg, maintenance dose of 60 μg
2. Loading dose of 60 μg, maintenance dose of 60 μg

Dose levels will include subjects randomized to sham-procedure or treatment with ultevursen.

Official Title
A Double-Masked, Randomized, Controlled, Multiple-Dose Study to Evaluate the Efficacy, Safety, and Tolerability of Ultevursen in Subjects With Retinitis Pigmentosa (RP) Due to Mutations in Exon 13 of the USH2A Gene (Sirius)

Conditions
Retinitis Pigmentosa
Usher Syndrome Type 2
Deaf Blind
Retinal Disease
Eye Diseases
Eye Diseases, Hereditary
Eye Disorders Congenital
Vision Disorders

Intervention/treatment
Drug: Ultevursen
Other: Sham-procedure

Other Study ID Numbers
PQ-421a-003
2021-002729-74 (EudraCT Number)

Study Start (Actual)
2021-12-08

Primary Completion (Estimated)
2024-12

Study Completion (Estimated)
2024-12

Enrollment (Estimated)
81

Study Type
Interventional

Phase
Phase 2 Phase 3

United States
California Locations

San Diego, California, United States, 92093-0946
Shiley Eye Institute - UC San Diego

San Francisco, California, United States, 94158
University of California, San Francisco

Florida Locations

Miami, Florida, United States, 33136
University of Miami, Bascom Palmer Eye Institute

Georgia Locations

Atlanta, Georgia, United States, 30322
Emory Eye Center

Maryland Locations
Baltimore, Maryland, United States, 21287
Wilmer Eye Institute, Johns Hopkins Hospital
Massachusetts Locations
Boston, Massachusetts, United States, 02114
Center for Clinical Research Operations, Massachusetts Eye and Ear
Michigan Locations
Ann Arbor, Michigan, United States, 48105
University of Michigan, Kellogg Eye Center
New York Locations
New York, New York, United States, 10032
Columbia University
Texas Locations
Dallas, Texas, United States, 75231
Retina Foundation of the Southwest
Wisconsin Locations
Madison, Wisconsin, United States, 53705
University of Wisconsin - Madison
Germany

Tuebingen, Germany, 72076
Universitaetsklinikum Tuebingen Department für Augenheilkunde

Netherlands

Nijmegen, Netherlands, 6525 GA
RadboudUMC

Rotterdam, Netherlands, 3011 BH
Het Oogziekenhuis Rotterdam

United Kingdom

London, United Kingdom
Moorfields Eye Hospital

Oxford Locations

Headington, Oxford, United Kingdom, OX3 9DU
Oxford Eye Hospital

Inclusion Criteria

- Male or female, ≥18 years of age OR a minor (12 to <18 years) with permission from a parent or legal guardian. The lower age limit for pediatric populations is subject to local regulatory and ethics committee requirements.
- An adult willing to comply with the protocol, follow study instructions, attend study visits as required and willing and able to complete all study assessments. OR A minor able to complete all study assessments and comply with the protocol and has a parent or caregiver willing and able to follow study instructions, and attend study visits with the subject as required.
- Clinical presentation consistent with RP with Usher syndrome type 2 or nonsyndromic form of RP (NSRP), based on ophthalmic, audiologic, and vestibular examinations.
- A molecular diagnosis of homozygosity or compound heterozygosity for 1 or more pathogenic exon 13 mutations in the USH2A gene, based on genetic analysis at screening.
- BCVA between ≥30 and ≤68 letters (approximate Snellen equivalent 20/250–20/50) in the treatment eye using the mean BCVA reading at screening. Subjects with a mean BCVA between >68 and ≤73 letters will be allowed with documented historic evidence of a BCVA equivalent decline of >5 letters in both eyes.
- BCVA between ≥30 and ≤73 letters (approximate Snellen equivalent 20/250–20/40) in the contralateral eye (CE), using the mean BCVA reading at Screening.
- A difference in mean BCVA readings at Screening between the TE and CE of ≤10 letters (based on ETDRS). BCVA differences between eyes that are greater than 10 letters may be allowed however, the Investigator should discuss the case with the Medical Monitor.
- Stable BCVA in the TE and CE, defined as two separate BCVA measurements at Screening that fall within ≤5 letters for each respective eye.
- A visible EZ layer on SD-OCT in the TE, as determined by the Investigator.
- No limitations to SD-OCT image collection that would prevent high quality, reliable images from being obtained in both eyes, as determined by the Investigator.
- Reliable BCVA, perimetry, and other measurements in both eyes, as described in the Study Reference Manual and Imaging Manual and determined by the Investigator.
- No visually significant ocular media opacities and adequate pupillary dilation to permit good quality retinal imaging in both eyes, as assessed by the Investigator.

Exclusion Criteria

- Presence of additional nonexon 13 USH2A pathogenic mutation(s) on the USH2A allele carrying the exon 13 mutation in subjects who have monoallelic exon-13 mutations.
- Presence of nonexon 13 USH2A pathogenic mutation(s) on both USH2A alleles in subjects who have biallelic exon 13 mutations.

- Presence of pathogenic mutations in genes (other than the USH2A gene) associated with Usher syndrome Type 2 or NSRP, or other inherited retinal degenerative diseases or syndromes. Note: The confirmed presence of homozygous or compound heterozygous known disease-causing mutations in other genes involved in recessive retinal dystrophies (RD), or the confirmed presence of known disease-causing mutations in genes involved in dominant or X-linked retinal dystrophies is exclusionary.
- Presence of any significant ocular (in either eye) or nonocular disease/disorder (or medication and/or laboratory test abnormalities) which, in the opinion of the Investigator and with concurrence of the Medical Monitor, may either put the subject at risk because of participation in the study, may influence the results of the study, or the subject's ability to participate in the study. This includes but is not limited to a subject who has uncontrolled cystoid macular edema (CME). CME is permissible if stable for 3 months (with or without treatment). Past CME is permissible if resolved for more than 1 month.
- History or presence of ocular herpetic diseases (including herpes simplex virus, varicella zoster or cytomegalovirus) in either eye.
- Presence of any active ocular infection in either eye.
- Presence of any of the following lens opacities in the study eye: cortical opacity ≥+2, posterior subcapsular opacity ≥+2, or a nuclear sclerosis ≥+2, and which are: (1) clinically significant in the opinion of the Investigator, (2) would adequately prevent clinical and photographic evaluation of the retina.
- History of amblyopia in either eye that resulted in significant vision loss, in the opinion of the Investigator.
- Receipt within 3 months prior to Screening of any intraocular or periocular surgery (including refractive surgery), or an IVT injection or planned intraocular surgery or procedure in either eye during the course of the study. For YAG laser treatment of a posterior capsular opacity, receipt within 1 month prior to Screening or planned procedure in either eye during the course of the study.
- Current treatment or treatment within the past 12 months with therapies known to influence the immune system (including but not limited to steroid implants, cytostatics, interferons, tumor necrosis factor (TNF)-binding proteins, drugs acting on immunophilins, or antibodies with known impact on the immune system). Subjects that have been treated with systemic steroids within the past 12 months or that require intermittent use of topical steroids may be considered for inclusion following approval by the Medical Monitor.
- A history of glaucoma or an IOP greater than 21 mmHg in either eye that is not controlled with medication or surgery. IOP measurements between 21 and 24 mmHg may be allowed; however, the Investigator should discuss the case with the Medical Monitor.
- Use of any investigational drug or device within 90 days or 5 half-lives preceding the first dose of study medication, whichever is longer, or plans to participate in another study of an investigational drug or device during the course of the study.
- Any prior treatment with genetic or stem-cell therapy for ocular or nonocular disease.

- History of malignancy within 2 years prior to Screening, except adequately treated squamous or basal cell carcinoma of the skin or carcinoma in situ of the cervix that has been successfully treated.
- Known hypersensitivity to antisense oligonucleotides or any constituents of the injection.
- Pregnant and breastfeeding subjects. Females of childbearing potential and males must comply with using highly effective methods of contraception as defined in the protocol. Women of nonchildbearing potential may be included without the use of adequate birth control.

Ages Eligible for Study
12 Years and older (Child, Adult, Older Adult)

Sexes Eligible for Study
All

Accepts Healthy Volunteers
No

- Primary Purpose: Treatment
- Allocation: Randomized
- Interventional Model: Parallel Assignment
- Interventional Model Description:
- Double-masked, randomized, controlled, multiple-dose study. Subjects will be randomized to one of three treatment groups:

  - Group 1: Ultevursen 180/60 μg (180 μg loading dose administered on Day 1, 60 μg maintenance dose administered at Month 3 and every 6 months thereafter)
  - Group 2: Ultevursen 60/60 μg (60 μg loading dose administered on Day 1, 60 μg maintenance dose administered at Month 3 and every 6 months thereafter; n = 27)
  - Group 3: Sham-procedure (administered on Day 1, Month 3, and every 6 months thereafter; n = 27)

- Masking: Quadruple (Participant Care Provider Investigator Outcomes Assessor)
- Masking Description: Subject, site staff (study coordinator, imaging technician, etc.) and Investigator will be completely masked. Physician performing IVT and post-IVT monitoring will know if subject is receiving sham or treatment, but will be masked to the dose level. Pharmacist is the only site staff that will be completely unmasked.

Arms and interventions

Participant group/arm	Intervention/treatment
Experimental: Ultevursen 180/60 μg 180 μg loading dose administered on Day 1, 60 μg maintenance dose administered at month 3 and every 6 months thereafter	Drug: Ultevursen • RNA antisense oligonucleotide for intravitreal injection • Other names: – RNA antisense oligonucleotide for intravitreal injection
Experimental: Ultevursen 60/60 μg 60 μg loading dose administered on Day 1, 60 μg maintenance dose administered at month 3 and every 6 months thereafter	Drug: Ultevursen • RNA antisense oligonucleotide for intravitreal injection • Other names – RNA antisense oligonucleotide for intravitreal injection
Sham comparator: sham-procedure Sham-procedure (no experimental drug administered) on day 1, month 3, and every 6 months thereafter	Other: Sham-procedure • Sham-procedure (no experimental drug administered)

Primary outcome measures

Outcome measure	Measure description	Time frame
Mean change from baseline in BCVA	Mean change from baseline in best corrected visual acuity(BCVA) based on the Early Treatment Diabetic Retinopathy Study (ETDRS) chart	18 months of treatment versus sham-procedure

Secondary outcome measures

Outcome measure	Measure description	Time frame
Proportion of patients who maintain vision defined by BCVA loss less than 15 Letters (ETDRS)	Proportion of patients who maintain vision defined by BCVA loss less than 15 letters based on ETDRS	27 months
Change from baseline in other analyses of BCVA	Change from baseline in other analyses of BCVA	27 months
Change from baseline in ellipsoid zone (EZ) area and width as imaged by spectral domain optical coherence tomography (SD-OCT)	Change from baseline in ellipsoid zone (EZ) area and width as imaged by spectral domain optical coherence tomography (SD-OCT)	27 months
Change from baseline in Low Luminance Visual Acuity (LLVA)	Change from baseline in Low Luminance Visual Acuity (LLVA)	27 months
Change from baseline in Microperimetry	Change from baseline in Microperimetry	27 months
Change from baseline in Full-field Stimulus Threshold (FST)	Change from baseline in Full-field Stimulus Threshold (FST)	27 months
Change from baseline in PRO measures	As assessed by the Veteran Affairs Low Vision Visual Functioning Questionnaire (VA LV VFQ-20), Patient Global Impressions of Severity (PGI-S) and Patient Global Impressions of Change (PGI-C)	27 months
Ocular and nonocular adverse events (AEs)	Ocular and nonocular adverse events (AEs)	27 months
Cmax of ultevursen in serum	Maximum concentration (Cmax) of ultevursen in serum	27 months

Sponsor
ProQR Therapeutics

Collaborators
No information provided

Investigators
Study Director: ProQR Medical Monitor, ProQR Therapeutics
Study Director: ProQR Clinical Trial Manager, ProQR Therapeutics

General Publications
No publications available

Results Submitted

Chapter 18
Not Yet Recruiting Studies

China

Clinical Trials of Continuous Oxygen Therapy Combined With Blue Light Deprivation in the Treatment of Retinitis Pigmentosa

ClinicalTrials.gov ID NCT02465749

Sponsor Sun Yat-Sen University
Information provided by Qianying Gao, Sun Yat-Sen University (Responsible Party)
Last Update Posted on 2015-06-08
Study Overview

Brief Summary
The purpose of this study is to investigate the role of continuous oxygen therapy combined with blue light deprivation in prevention and control of retinitis pigmentosa, in order to find a new strategy of treatment for retinitis pigmentosa.

Detailed Description
Retinitis pigmentosa (RP) is one of the major causes of blindness in ocular diseases. Up to now, the etiology of RP remained unclear, and there are no effective therapeutic methods.

Several studies had showed that the retina of RP may be anoxic, and oxygen therapy, such as hyperbaric oxygen (hyperbaric oxygen, HBO) treatment, had shown a definite effect on RP. The investigators' previous research also found that the retinal vessel oxygen saturation in patients with RP who were older than 40 years were significantly lower than normal controls, suggesting that oxygen may play an important role in the development of RP. Besides, many studies have revealed that blue light could damage retina pigment epithelium cells and

J. N. Weiss, *Clinical Trials in Retinitis Pigmentosa Treatment*,
https://doi.org/10.1007/978-3-031-58799-3_18

photoreceptor cell specially. Therefore, investigators will combine continuous oxygen therapy and blue light deprivation therapy in the treatment for RP in this study, in order to find a new strategy of treatment for RP.

Official Title
Clinical Trials of Continuous Oxygen Therapy Combined With Blue Light Deprivation in the Treatment of Retinitis Pigmentosa

Conditions
Retinitis Pigmentosa

Intervention/Treatment
Drug: Continuous oxygen
Device: blue light-absorbing sunglasses
Drug: Compound thrombosis capsule sig: 1.5 g/tid
Drug: Ginkgo biloba pills sig: 300 mg/tid
Drug: Vitamin B sig: 10 mg/tid
Drug: Vitamin AD sig: 1 tablet/tid

Other Study ID Numbers
ZOC20150503

Study Start
2015-05

Primary Completion (Estimated)
2025-06

Study Completion (Estimated)
2025-06

Enrollment (Estimated)
404

Study Type
Interventional

Phase
Early Phase 1

Study Contact
Name: Qianying Gao, PHD
Phone Number: 13751829105/18922103820
Email: gaoqy@mail.sysu.edu.cn
China
Guangdong Locations
Guangzhou, Guangdong, China, 510060
State Key Laboratory of Ophthalmology, Zhongshan Ophthalmic Center, Sun Yat-Sen University

Contact

Qianying Qao, PHD
13751829105/18922103820gaoqy@mail.sysu.edu.cn

Eligibility Criteria

Description

Inclusion Criteria

- Severe patients with RP who meet the following criteria: (1) the EDTRS visual acuity of the good eye <0.3 (low vision) and (2) the radius of central visual field <10° (low vision)
- Age range from 18 to 60 years old, sex unlimited
- Able to adhere to treatment for more than 12 months
- Willing to participate in this trial, and sign the informed consent

Exclusion Criteria

- Serious opacity of cornea, lens, or vitreous body which can't have clear fundus examination
- Patients with severe systemic diseases who was unable to tolerate the examinations, such as heart failure, respiratory failure, sepsis, severe anemia, kidney disease, history of eye surgery, and so on
- Patients who was unable to tolerate oxygen treatment, such as severe pulmonary edema, deformity of the respiratory tract, respiratory tract infection, tuberculosis, patients with pregnancy, and so on

Ages Eligible for Study

18–60 Years (Adult)

Sexes Eligible for Study

All

Accepts Healthy Volunteers

No

Design Details

Primary Purpose: Treatment
Allocation: Randomized
Interventional Model: Parallel Assignment
Masking: None (Open Label)

Arms and interventions

Participant group/arm	Intervention/treatment
Experimental: Continuous oxygen Continuous oxygen intake and routine drug treatment	Drug: Continuous oxygen • Continuous oxygen intake at a concentration of 93 ± 3%, 3 L/min flow-rate, 2 h/bid, 5 days a week Drug: compound thrombosis capsule sig: 1.5 g/tid • Compound thrombosis capsule sig: 1.5 g/tid Drug: Ginkgo biloba pills sig: 300 mg/tid • Ginkgo biloba pills sig: 300 mg/tid Drug: Vitamin B sig: 10 mg/tid • Vitamin B sig: 10 mg/tid Drug: Vitamin AD sig: 1 tablet/tid • Vitamin AD sig: 1 tablet/tid

Experimental: Blue Light Deprivation Wearing blue light-absorbing sunglasses at daily time and routine drug treatment	Device: blue light-absorbing sunglasses • Wearing blue light-absorbing sunglasses at daily time Drug: Compound thrombosis capsule sig: 1.5 g/tid • Compound thrombosis capsule sig: 1.5 g/tid Drug: Ginkgo biloba pills sig: 300 mg/tid • Ginkgo biloba pills sig: 300 mg/tid Drug: Vitamin B sig: 10 mg/tid • Vitamin B sig: 10 mg/tid Drug: Vitamin AD sig: 1 tablet/tid • Vitamin AD sig: 1 tablet/tid
Experimental: Continuous oxygen therapy combined with blue light deprivation Continuous oxygen intake, wearing blue light-absorbing sunglasses at daily time and routine drug treatment	Drug: Continuous oxygen • Continuous oxygen intake at a concentration of 93 ± 3%, 3 L/min flow-rate, 2 h/bid, 5 days a week Device: blue light-absorbing sunglasses • Wearing blue light-absorbing sunglasses at daily time Drug: Compound thrombosis capsule sig: 1.5 g/tid • Compound thrombosis capsule sig: 1.5 g/tid Drug: Ginkgo biloba pills sig: 300 mg/tid • Ginkgo biloba pills sig: 300 mg/tid Drug: Vitamin B sig: 10 mg/tid • Vitamin B sig: 10 mg/tid Drug: Vitamin AD sig: 1 tablet/tid • Vitamin AD sig: 1 tablet/tid
Other: control Routine drug treatment	Drug: Compound thrombosis capsule sig: 1.5 g/tid • Compound thrombosis capsule sig: 1.5 g/tid Drug: Ginkgo biloba pills sig: 300 mg/tid; • Ginkgo biloba pills sig: 300 mg/tid; Drug: Vitamin B sig: 10 mg/tid • Vitamin B sig: 10 mg/tid Drug: Vitamin AD sig: 1 tablet/tid • Vitamin AD sig: 1 tablet/tid

Primary outcome measures

Outcome measure	Measure description	Time frame
The percentage of patients preserved 80% of the initial visual acuity at 5 years follow-up		At 5 years follow-up

Secondary outcome measures

Outcome measure	Measure description	Time frame
ERG B-wave mean values		At 5 years follow-up
Change of visual field	Visual field	At 5 years follow-up
Fundus changes of fluorescence fundus angiography		At 5 years follow-up
Retinal vessel oxygen saturation	Retinal oximetry	At 5 years follow-up
Intraocular pressure		At 1, 2, 3, 4, and 5 years follow-up
Blood pressure		At 1, 2, 3, 4, and 5 years follow-up
Finger pulse oxygen saturation	Finger pulse oximetry	At 1, 2, 3, 4, and 5 years follow-up
The mutant genes of retinitis pigmentosa	Gene screening	At admission

Sponsor
Sun Yat-Sen University

Collaborators
Zhujiang Hospital
Sun Yat-Sen Memorial Hospital of Sun Yat-Sen University
Guangzhou Jeeyor Medical Research Co., Ltd.

Investigators
Principal Investigator: Qianying Gao, PHD, State Key Laboratory of Ophthalmology, Zhongshan Ophthalmic Center, Sun Yat-sen University

General Publications
No publications available

Appendix: Tables

See Tables A.1, A.2, A.3, and A.4.

J. N. Weiss, *Clinical Trials in Retinitis Pigmentosa Treatment*,
https://doi.org/10.1007/978-3-031-58799-3

Table A.1 Stem cell completed studies

	UNITED STATES	BRAZIL	TURKEY
NUMBER OF COMPLETED STUDIES	3	2	1
CORPORATE	3		
UNIVERSITY/HOSPITAL		2	1
NO SUPPORT			
DELIVERY METHOD	Intravitreal	Intravitreal	Suprachoroidal
RESULTS	Yes	No	No
BONE MARROW		2	
IPSC			
ADIPOSE			
PROPRIETARY	3		
UMBILICAL			1
EMBRYONIC			
WHARTONS			

Table A.2 Stem cell recruiting studies

	UNITED STATES	ASIA	MIDDLE EAST	CARIBBEAN/SOUTH AMERICA
NUMBER OF STUDIES	4	1	1	1
CORPORATE	1		1	
UNIVERSITY/HOSPITAL/NEI	2	1		
NO SUPPORT	1			1
BONE MARROW	2			
IPSC				
ADIPOSE				
PROPRIETARY	2			
UMBILICAL		1	1	1
EMBRYONIC				
WHARTONS				

Table A.3 Gene completed studies

	UNITED STATES	INDIA	SAUDI ARABIA
NUMBER OF STUDIES	3	1	1
CORPORATE	3	1	
UNIVERSITY/HOSPITAL/NEI			1
NO SUPPORT			
RESULTS	0	0	1

Table A.4 Gene recruiting studies

	UNITED STATES/EUROPE/ISRAEL	CHINA
NUMBER OF STUDIES	6	1
CORPORATE	6	1
UNIVERSITY/HOSPITAL		
NO SUPPORT		

References

Retinitis Pigmentosa

1. Hartong DT, Berson EL, Dryja TP. Retinitis pigmentosa. Lancet. 2006;368(9549):1795–809.
2. Brooks BP, Jeffrey B. Methodological insights for randomized clinical trials of retinitis pigmentosa: lessons learned from a trial of valproic acid. JAMA Ophthalmol. 2018;136(8):857–8.
3. Newell FW. Clinical trials and retinitis pigmentosa. Am J Ophthalmol. 1978;85(5):720–1.
4. Macdonald AE, McKenzie KG. Sympathectomy for Retinitis Pigmentosa. Trans Am Ophthalmol Soc. 1934;32:172–90.
5. Hoffman DR, Hughbanks-Wheaton DK, Spencer R, Fish GE, Pearson NS, Wang YZ, et al. Docosahexaenoic acid slows visual field progression in X-linked retinitis pigmentosa: ancillary outcomes of the DHAX trial. Invest Ophthalmol Vis Sci. 2015;56(11):6646–53.
6. Chatzinoff A, Nelson E, Stahl N, Clahane A. Eleven-CIS vitamin A in the treatment of retinitis pigmentosa. A negative study. Arch Ophthalmol. 1968;80(4):417–9.
7. Dagnelie G, Zorge IS, McDonald TM. Lutein improves visual function in some patients with retinal degeneration: a pilot study via the Internet. Optometry. 2000;71(3):147–64.
8. Brito-Garcia N, Del Pino-Sedeno T, Trujillo-Martin MM, Coco RM, Rodriguez de la Rua E, Del Cura-Gonzalez I, et al. Effectiveness and safety of nutritional supplements in the treatment of hereditary retinal dystrophies: a systematic review. Eye. 2017;31(2):273–85.
9. Berson EL, Rosner B, Sandberg MA, Hayes KC, Nicholson BW, Weigel-DiFranco C, et al. A randomized trial of vitamin A and vitamin E supplementation for retinitis pigmentosa. Arch Ophthalmol. 1993;111(6):761–72.
10. Berson EL, Rosner B, Sandberg MA, Weigel-DiFranco C, Moser A, Brockhurst RJ, et al. Clinical trial of docosahexaenoic acid in patients with retinitis pigmentosa receiving vitamin A treatment. Arch Ophthalmol. 2004;122(9):1297–305.
11. Berson EL, Rosner B, Sandberg MA, Weigel-DiFranco C, Brockhurst RJ, Hayes KC, et al. Clinical trial of lutein in patients with retinitis pigmentosa receiving vitamin A. Arch Ophthalmol. 2010;128(4):403–11.
12. Berson EL, Sandberg MA, Rosner B, Birch DG, Hanson AH. Natural course of retinitis pigmentosa over a three-year interval. Am J Ophthalmol. 1985;99(3):240–51.
13. Andreasson SO, Sandberg MA, Berson EL. Narrow-band filtering for monitoring low- amplitude cone electroretinograms in retinitis pigmentosa. Am J Ophthalmol. 1988;105(5):500–3.
14. Berson EL. Long-term visual prognoses in patients with retinitis pigmentosa: the Ludwig von Sallmann lecture. Exp Eye Res. 2007;85(1):7–14.

J. N. Weiss, *Clinical Trials in Retinitis Pigmentosa Treatment*,
https://doi.org/10.1007/978-3-031-58799-3

15. Berson EL, Retinitis pigmentosa. The Friedenwald lecture. Invest Ophthalmol Vis Sci. 1993;34(5):1659–76.
16. Norton EW. A randomized trial of vitamin A and vitamin E supplementation for retinitis pigmentosa. Arch Ophthalmol. 1993;111(11):1460; author reply 3–5.
17. Marmor MF. A randomized trial of vitamin A and vitamin E supplementation for retinitis pigmentosa. Arch Ophthalmol. 1993;111(11):1460–1; author reply 3–5.
18. Clowes DD. A randomized trial of vitamin A and vitamin E supplementation for retinitis pigmentosa. Arch Ophthalmol. 1993;111(11):1461–2; author reply 2–5.
19. Massof RW, Finkelstein D. Supplemental vitamin A retards loss of ERG amplitude in retinitis pigmentosa. Arch Ophthalmol. 1993;111(6):751–4.
20. Massof RW, Fishman GA. How strong is the evidence that nutritional supplements slow the progression of retinitis pigmentosa? Arch Ophthalmol. 2010;128(4):493–5.
21. Gamel JW, Barr CC. A randomized trial of vitamin A and vitamin E supplementation for retinitis pigmentosa. Arch Ophthalmol. 1993;111(11):1462–3.
22. Wan A, Place E, Pierce EA, Comander J. Characterizing variants of unknown significance in rhodopsin: a functional genomics approach. Hum Mutat. 2019;40(8):1127–44.
23. Li T, Sandberg MA, Pawlyk BS, Rosner B, Hayes KC, Dryja TP, et al. Effect of vitamin A supplementation on rhodopsin mutants threonine-17 → methionine and proline-347 → serine in transgenic mice and in cell cultures. Proc Natl Acad Sci USA. 1998;95(20):11933–8.
24. Cui X, Kim HJ, Cheng CH, Jenny LA, Lima de Carvalho JR, Chang YJ, et al. Long-term vitamin A supplementation in a preclinical mouse model for RhoD190N-associated retinitis pigmentosa. Hum Mol Genet. 2022;31(14):2438–51.
25. Krasovec T, Kobal N, Sustar Habjan M, Volk M, Hawlina M, Fakin A. Correlation between the serum concentration of vitamin A and disease severity in patients carrying p.G90D in RHO, the most frequent gene associated with dominant retinitis pigmentosa: implications for therapy with vitamin A. Int J Mol Sci. 2023;24(1):780.
26. Consugar MB, Navarro-Gomez D, Place EM, Bujakowska KM, Sousa ME, Fonseca-Kelly ZD, et al. Panel-based genetic diagnostic testing for inherited eye diseases is highly accurate and reproducible, and more sensitive for variant detection, than exome sequencing. Genet Med. 2015;17(4):253–61.
27. Zampaglione E, Maher M, Place EM, Wagner NE, DiTroia S, Chao KR, et al. The importance of automation in genetic diagnosis: Lessons from analyzing an inherited retinal degeneration cohort with the Mendelian Analysis Toolkit (MATK). Genet Med. 2022;24(2):332–43.
28. Berson EL, Weigel-DiFranco C, Rosner B, Gaudio AR, Sandberg MA. Association of Vitamin A supplementation with disease course in children with retinitis pigmentosa. JAMA Ophthalmol. 2018;136(5):490–5.
29. Rahmani S, Comander J, DiFranco CW, Rosner B, Sandberg MA. A biomarker for disease course in patients with autosomal dominant retinitis pigmentosa due to RHO mutations. Invest Ophthalmol Vis Sci. 2016;57(12):1.
30. Sandberg MA, Rosner B, Weigel-DiFranco C, McGee TL, Dryja TP, Berson EL. Disease course in patients with autosomal recessive retinitis pigmentosa due to the USH2A gene. Invest Ophthalmol Vis Sci. 2008;49(12):5532–9.
31. Sandberg MA, Rosner B, Weigel-DiFranco C, Dryja TP, Berson EL. Disease course of patients with X-linked retinitis pigmentosa due to RPGR gene mutations. Invest Ophthalmol Vis Sci. 2007;48(3):1298–304.
32. Berson EL, Rosner B, Weigel-DiFranco C, Dryja TP, Sandberg MA. Disease progression in patients with dominant retinitis pigmentosa and rhodopsin mutations. Invest Ophthalmol Vis Sci. 2002;43(9):3027–36.
33. Hafler BP, Comander J, Weigel DiFranco C, Place EM, Pierce EA. Course of ocular function in PRPF31 retinitis pigmentosa. Semin Ophthalmol. 2016;31(1-2):49–52.
34. Jacobson SG, Marmor MF, Kemp CM, Knighton RW. SWS (blue) cone hypersensitivity in a newly identified retinal degeneration. Invest Ophthalmol Vis Sci. 1990;31(5):827–38.

35. Sajovic J, Meglic A, Glavac D, Markelj S, Hawlina M, Fakin A. The role of Vitamin A in retinal diseases. Int J Mol Sci. 2022;23(3):1014.
36. Comander J, Weigel-DiFranco C, Sandberg MA, Berson EL. Visual function in carriers of X-linked retinitis pigmentosa. Ophthalmology. 2015;122(9):1899–906.
37. Daiger SP, Bowne SJ, Sullivan LS, Branham K, Wheaton DK, Jones KD, et al. Molecular findings in families with an initial diagnose of autosomal dominant retinitis pigmentosa (adRP). Adv Exp Med Biol. 2018;1074:237–45.
38. Sengillo JD, Cabral T, Schuerch K, Duong J, Lee W, Boudreault K, et al. Electroretinography reveals difference in cone function between syndromic and nonsyndromic USH2A patients. Sci Rep. 2017;7(1):11170.
39. Pierrache LH, Hartel BP, van Wijk E, Meester-Smoor MA, Cremers FP, de Baere E, et al. Visual prognosis in USH2A-associated retinitis pigmentosa is worse for patients with usher syndrome type IIa than for those with nonsyndromic retinitis pigmentosa. Ophthalmology. 2016;123(5):1151–60.
40. Birch DG, Cheng P, Duncan JL, Ayala AR, Maguire MG, Audo I, et al. The RUSH2A study: best-corrected visual acuity, full-field electroretinography amplitudes, and full-field stimulus thresholds at baseline. Transl Vis Sci Technol. 2020;9(11):9.
41. Comander J, Bujakowska KM, Pierce EA. Natural history of retinitis pigmentosa based on genotype, vitamin A/E supplementation, and an electroretinogram biomarker. JCI Insight. 2023;8(15):e167546. https://doi.org/10.1172/jci.insight.167546.

Luxturna

42. Steinkuller PG, Du L, Gilbert C, Foster A, Collins ML, Coats DK. Childhood blindness. J AAPOS. 1999;3(1):26–32.
43. Sharif W, Sharif Z. Leber's congenital amaurosis and the role of gene therapy in congenital retinal disorders. Int J Ophthalmol. 2017;10(3):480–4.
44. Samardzija M, Barben M, Geiger P, Grimm C. The consequences of hypomorphic RPE65 for rod and cone photoreceptors. Adv Exp Med Biol. 2016;854:341–6.
45. Reape K, Chung D, Schaefer G, et al. Natural history of individuals with retinal degeneration due to biallelic mutations in the RPE65 gene. Paper presented at: ARVO2017; Baltimore, MD.
46. Sparrow JR, Hicks D, Hamel CP. The retinal pigment epithelium in health and disease. Curr Mol Med. 2010;10(9):802–23.
47. Astuti GD, Bertelsen M, Preising MN, et al. Comprehensive genotyping reveals RPE65 as the most frequently mutated gene in Leber congenital amaurosis in Denmark. Eur J Hum Genet. 2016;24(7):1071–9.
48. Kumaran N, Moore AT, Weleber RG, Michaelides M. Leber congenital amaurosis/early-onset severe retinal dystrophy: clinical features, molecular genetics and therapeutic interventions. Br J Ophthalmol. 2017;101(9):1147–54.
49. Chung D, Wellman J, et al. The natural history of disease progression in patients with RPE65-mediated inherited retinal dystrophy. Invest Ophthalmol Vis Sci. 2016;2017:6588. http://iovs.arvojournals.org/article.aspx?articleid=2564400.
50. Spark Therapeutics Inc. FDA Advisory Committee Briefing Document Spark Therapeutics, Inc. Luxturnatm (voretigene neparvovec). In: Meeting of the cellular, tissue, and gene therapies advisory committee meeting. 2017. https://www.fda.gov/downloads/AdvisoryCommittees/CommitteesMeetingMaterials/BloodVac cinesandOtherBiologics/CellularTissueandGeneTherapiesAdvisoryCommittee/UCM579300.pdf. Accessed 12 October 2017.
51. den Hollander AI, Roepman R, Koenekoop RK, Cremers FP. Leber congenital amaurosis: genes, proteins and disease mechanisms. Prog Retin Eye Res. 2008;27(4):391–419.

52. Weleber R, Francis P, Trzupek K, Beattie C. Leber Congenital Amaurosis. In: Pagon RA, Ardinger HH, et al., editors. GeneReviews. Seattle: University of Washington; 2013.
53. Paunescu K, Wabbels B, Preising MN, Lorenz B. Longitudinal and cross-sectional study of patients with early-onset severe retinal dystrophy associated with RPE65 mutations. Graefes Arch Clin Exp Ophthalmol. 2005;243(5):417–26.
54. Alkharashi M, Fulton AB. Available evidence on leber congenital amaurosis and gene therapy. Semin Ophthalmol. 2017;32(1):14–21.
55. Chung DC, Traboulsi EI. Leber congenital amaurosis: clinical correlations with genotypes, gene therapy trials update, and future directions. J AAPOS. 2009;13(6):587–92.
56. Walia S, Fishman GA, Jacobson SG, et al. Visual acuity in patients with Leber's congenital amaurosis and early childhood-onset retinitis pigmentosa. Ophthalmology. 2010;117(6):1190–8.
57. Jacobson SG, Aleman TS, Cideciyan AV, et al. Defining the residual vision in leber congenital amaurosis caused by RPE65 mutations. Invest Ophthalmol Vis Sci. 2009;50(5):2368–75.
58. Testa F, Melillo P, Di Lorio V, et al. Chromatic pupillometry as an objective outcome to evaluate effects of Voretigene Neparvovec treatment in patients with RPE65-related inherited retinal dystrophies. Presented at: Association for Research in Vision and Ophthalmology (ARVO) 2023 Annual Meeting. April 23-27, 2023; New Orleans, LA. Abstract #5445.
59. Kiraly P, Cottriall C, Taylor LJ, et al. Functional outcomes and adverse effects of voretigene neparvovec for biallelic RPE65-mediated inherited retinal dystrophies in a cohort of patients from a single centre. Presented at: Association for Research in Vision and Ophthalmology (ARVO) 2023 Annual Meeting. April 23-27, 2023; New Orleans, LA. Abstract #801 – C0402.
60. Hertens L, Cauwenbergh CV, den Broeck FV, et al. Results of Belgian patients with RPE65-related inherited retinal dystrophy 6 months after treatment with voretigene neparvovec. Presented at: Association for Research in Vision and Ophthalmology (ARVO) 2023 Annual Meeting. April 23-27, 2023; New Orleans, LA. Abstract #762 – C0363.
61. Voretigene Neparvovec for Biallelic RPE65-Mediated retinal disease: effectiveness and value final evidence report February 14, 2018 ICER Institute for Clinical and Economic Review.

Stem Cells

62. Caplan AI. Adult mesenchymal stem cells for tissue engineering versus regenerative medicine. J Cell Physiol. 2007;213:341–7.
63. Da Silva Meirelles L, Cesar Chagastelles P, Beyer Nardi N. Mesenchymal stem cells reside in virtually all post-natal organs and tissues. J Cell Sci. 2006;119:2204–13.
64. Crisan M, Yap S, Casteilla L. A perivascular origin for mesenchymal stem cells in multiple human organs. Cell Stem Cell. 2008;3:301–13.
65. Guimarães-Camboa N, Cattaneo P, Sun Y, et al. Pericytes of multiple organs do not behave as mesenchymal stem cells. Cell Stem Cell. 2017;20:345–59.
66. Caplan AI, Correa D. The MSC: an injury drugstore cell stem. Cell. 2011;9:11–5.
67. Caplan AI. Mesenchymal stem cells: time to change the name! Stem Cells Transl Med. 2017;6:1445–51.
68. Le Blanc K, Rasmusson I, Sundberg B. Treatment of severe acute graft-versus-host disease with third party haploidentical mesenchymal stem cells. Lancet. 2004;363:1439–41.
69. Carvalho AÉS, Sousa MRR, Alencar-Silva T, et al. Mesenchymal stem cells immunomodulation: the road to IFN-γ licensing and the path ahead. Cytokine Growth Factor Rev. 2019;47:32–42.
70. Klingemann H, Matzilevich D, Marchand J. Mesenchymal stem cells - sources and clinical applications. Transfus Med Hemother. 2008;35:2.

71. Hass R, Kasper C, Böhm S, et al. Different populations and sources of human mesenchymal stem cells (MSC): a comparison of adult and neonatal tissue-derived MSC. Cell Commun Signal. 2011;9:1–14.
72. Kim N, Cho SG. Clinical applications of mesenchymal stem cells. Korean J Intern Med. 2013;28:387.
73. Suchanek J, Soukup T, Visek B, et al. Dental pulp stem cells and their characterization. Biomed Pap. 2009;153:31–6.
74. Sivasubramaniyan K, Lehnen D, Ghazanfari R, et al. Phenotypic and functional heterogeneity of human bone marrow – and amnion-derived MSC subsets. Ann N Y Acad Sci. 2012;1266:94–106.
75. La Rocca G, Anzalone R, Corrao S, et al. Isolation and characterization of Oct-4 +/HLA-G + mesenchymal stem cells from human umbilical cord matrix: differentiation potential and detection of new markers. Histochem Cell Biol. 2009;131:267–82.
76. Vellasamy S, Sandrasaigaran P, Vidyadaran S, et al. Isolation and characterisation of mesenchymal stem cells derived from human placenta tissue. World J Stem Cells. 2012;4:53–61.
77. Wang AT, Feng Y, Jia HH, et al. Application of mesenchymal stem cell therapy for the treatment of osteoarthritis of the knee: a concise review. World J Stem Cells. 2019;11:222.
78. Vu Q, Xie K, Eckert M, et al. Meta-analysis of preclinical studies of mesenchymal stromal cells for ischemic stroke. Neurology. 2014;82:1277–86.
79. Tyndall A. Mesenchymal stromal cells and rheumatic disorders. Immunol Lett. 2015;168:201–7.
80. Kim J, Shapiro L, Flynn A. The clinical application of mesenchymal stem cells and cardiac stem cells as a therapy for cardiovascular disease. Pharmacol Ther. 2015;151:8–15.
81. Matthay MA, Goolaerts A, Howard JP, et al. Mesenchymal stem cells for acute lung injury: preclinical evidence. Crit Care Med. 2010;38(10):569–73.
82. Ozmert E, Arslan U. Management of retinitis pigmentosa via Wharton's jelly-derived mesenchymal stem cells or combination with magnovision: 3-year prospective results. Stem Cells Transl Med. 2023;12:631–50. https://doi.org/10.1093/stcltm/szad051.

Gene Therapy

83. Hu ML, Edwards TL, O'Hare F, Hickey DG, Wang JH, Liu Z, Ayton LN. Gene therapy for inherited retinal diseases: progress and possibilities. Clin Exp Optom. 2021;104(4):444–54. https://doi.org/10.1080/08164622.2021.1880863. Epub 2021 Mar 2. PMID: 33689657.
84. Rodrigues GA, Shalaev E, Karami TK, Cunningham J, Slater NKH, Rivers HM. Pharmaceutical development of AAV-based gene therapy products for the eye. Pharm Res. 2018;36(2):29. https://doi.org/10.1007/s11095-018-2554-7. PMID: 30591984; PMCID: PMC6308217.
85. High KA, Roncarolo MG. Gene therapy. N Engl J Med. 2019;381(5):455–64. https://doi.org/10.1056/NEJMra1706910. PMID: 31365802.
86. Ducloyer JB, Le Meur G, Cronin T, Adjali O, Weber M. Gene therapy for retinitis pigmentosa. Med Sci. 2020;36(6-7, 607):–615. https://doi.org/10.1051/medsci/2020095. Epub 2020 Jul 2. PMID: 32614312.
87. Dhurandhar D, Sahoo NK, Mariappan I, Narayanan R. Gene therapy in retinal diseases: a review. Indian J Ophthalmol. 2021;69(9):2257–65. https://doi.org/10.4103/ijo.IJO_3117_20. PMID: 34427196; PMCID: PMC8544052.
88. Britten-Jones AC, Jin R, Gocuk SA, Cichello E, O'Hare F, Hickey DG, Edwards TL, Ayton LN. The safety and efficacy of gene therapy treatment for monogenic retinal and optic nerve diseases: a systematic review. Genet Med. 2022;24(3):521–34. https://doi.org/10.1016/j.gim.2021.10.013. Epub 2021 Nov 30. PMID: 34906485.

89. Petit L, Khanna H, Punzo C. Advances in gene therapy for diseases of the eye. Hum Gene Ther. 2016;27(8):563–79. https://doi.org/10.1089/hum.2016.040. Epub 2016 Jun 13. PMID: 27178388; PMCID: PMC4991575.
90. Prado DA, Acosta-Acero M, Maldonado RS. Gene therapy beyond luxturna: a new horizon of the treatment for inherited retinal disease. Curr Opin Ophthalmol. 2020;31(3):147–54. https://doi.org/10.1097/ICU.0000000000000660. PMID: 32175942.
91. Botto C, Rucli M, Tekinsoy MD, Pulman J, Sahel JA, Dalkara D. Early and late stage gene therapy interventions for inherited retinal degenerations. Prog Retin Eye Res. 2022;86:100975. https://doi.org/10.1016/j.preteyeres.2021.100975. Epub 2021 May 29. PMID: 34058340.
92. Switonski M. Impact of gene therapy for canine monogenic diseases on the progress of preclinical studies. J Appl Genet. 2020;61(2):179–86. https://doi.org/10.1007/s13353-020-00554-8. Epub 2020 Mar 18. PMID: 32189222; PMCID: PMC7148265.

Optogenetics

93. Duebel J, Marazova K, Sahel JA. Optogenetics. Curr Opin Ophthalmol. 2015;26(3):226–32. https://doi.org/10.1097/ICU.0000000000000140. PMID: 25759964; PMCID: PMC5395664.
94. Liu W, Liu S, Li P, Yao K. Retinitis pigmentosa: progress in molecular pathology and biotherapeutical strategies. Int J Mol Sci. 2022;23(9):4883. https://doi.org/10.3390/ijms23094883. PMID: 35563274; PMCID: PMC9101511.
95. Bamberg E, Gärtner W, Trauner D. Introduction: optogenetics and photopharmacology. Chem Rev. 2018;118(21):10627–8. https://doi.org/10.1021/acs.chemrev.8b00483. PMID: 30424609.
96. Fenner BJ, Tan TE, Barathi AV, Tun SBB, Yeo SW, Tsai ASH, Lee SY, Cheung CMG, Chan CM, Mehta JS, Teo KYC. Gene-based therapeutics for inherited retinal diseases. Front Genet. 2022;12:794805. https://doi.org/10.3389/fgene.2021.794805. PMID: 35069693; PMCID: PMC8782148.
97. Ziccardi L, Cordeddu V, Gaddini L, Matteucci A, Parravano M, Malchiodi-Albedi F, Varano M. Gene therapy in retinal dystrophies. Int J Mol Sci. 2019;20(22):5722. https://doi.org/10.3390/ijms20225722. PMID: 31739639; PMCID: PMC6888000.
98. Harris AR, Gilbert F. Restoring vision using optogenetics without being blind to the risks. Graefes Arch Clin Exp Ophthalmol. 2022;260(1):41–5. https://doi.org/10.1007/s00417-021-05477-6. Epub 2021 Nov 1. PMID: 34724112; PMCID: PMC8558540.
99. Sahel JA, Boulanger-Scemama E, Pagot C, Arleo A, Galluppi F, Martel JN, Esposti SD, Delaux A, de Saint Aubert JB, de Montleau C, Gutman E, Audo I, Duebel J, Picaud S, Dalkara D, Blouin L, Taiel M, Roska B. Partial recovery of visual function in a blind patient after optogenetic therapy. Nat Med. 2021;27(7):1223–9. https://doi.org/10.1038/s41591-021-01351-4. Epub 2021 May 24. PMID: 34031601.
100. Losi A, Gardner KH, Möglich A. Blue-light receptors for optogenetics. Chem Rev. 2018;118(21):10659–709. https://doi.org/10.1021/acs.chemrev.8b00163. Epub 2018 Jul 9. PMID: 29984995; PMCID: PMC6500593.
101. Tomita H, Sugano E. Optogenetics-mediated gene therapy for retinal diseases. Adv Exp Med Biol. 2021;1293:535–43. https://doi.org/10.1007/978-981-15-8763-4_37. PMID: 33398840

Other Treatments

102. Chan HH, Lam HI, Choi KY, Li SZ, Lakshmanan Y, Yu WY, Chang RC, Lai JS, So KF. Delay of cone degeneration in retinitis pigmentosa using a 12-month treatment with Lycium barbarum supplement. J Ethnopharmacol. 2019;236:336–44. https://doi.org/10.1016/j.jep.2019.03.023. Epub 2019 Mar 12. PMID: 30877066.
103. Birch DG, Bernstein PS, Iannacone A, Pennesi ME, Lam BL, Heckenlively J, Csaky K, Hartnett ME, Winthrop KL, Jayasundera T, Hughbanks-Wheaton DK, Warner J, Yang P, Fish GE, Teske MP, Sklaver NL, Erker L, Chegarnov E, Smith T, Wahle A, VanVeldhuisen PC, McCormack J, Lindblad R, Bramer S, Rose S, Zilliox P, Francis PJ, Weleber RG. Effect of oral valproic acid vs placebo for vision loss in patients with autosomal dominant retinitis pigmentosa: a randomized phase 2 multicenter placebo-controlled clinical trial. JAMA Ophthalmol. 2018;136(8):849–56. https://doi.org/10.1001/jamaophthalmol.2018.1171. Erratum in: JAMA Ophthalmol. 2018 Dec 1;136(12):1432. PMID: 29879277; PMCID: PMC6142953.
104. Dizdar Yigit D, Sevik MO, Şahin Ö. Transcorneal electrical stimulation therapy may have a stabilization effect on multifocal electroretinography for patients with retinitis pigmentosa. Retina. 2022;42(5):923–33. https://doi.org/10.1097/IAE.0000000000003386. PMID: 34923514.
105. Akiyama M, Ikeda Y, Yoshida N, Notomi S, Murakami Y, Hisatomi T, Enaida H, Ishibashi T. Therapeutic efficacy of topical unoprostone isopropyl in retinitis pigmentosa. Acta Ophthalmol. 2014;92(3):e229–34. https://doi.org/10.1111/aos.12293. PMID: 24868583.
106. Jolly JK, Wagner SK, Martus P, MacLaren RE, Wilhelm B, Webster AR, Downes SM, Charbel Issa P, Kellner U, Jägle H, Rüther K, Bertelsen M, Bragadóttir R, Prener Holtan J, van den Born LI, Sodi A, Virgili G, Gosheva M, Pach J, Zündorf I, Zrenner E, Gekeler F. Transcorneal electrical stimulation for the treatment of retinitis pigmentosa: a multicenter safety study of the OkuStim® system (TESOLA-Study). Ophthalmic Res. 2020;63(3):234–43. https://doi.org/10.1159/000505001. Epub 2019 Nov 26. PMID: 31775146.
107. Birch DG, Bennett LD, Duncan JL, Weleber RG, Pennesi ME. Long-term follow-up of patients with retinitis pigmentosa receiving intraocular ciliary neurotrophic factor implants. Am J Ophthalmol. 2016;170:10–4. https://doi.org/10.1016/j.ajo.2016.07.013. Epub 2016 Jul 25. PMID: 27457255; PMCID: PMC5056139.
108. Hoffman DR, Hughbanks-Wheaton DK, Pearson NS, Fish GE, Spencer R, Takacs A, Klein M, Locke KG, Birch DG. Four-year placebo-controlled trial of docosahexaenoic acid in X-linked retinitis pigmentosa (DHAX trial): a randomized clinical trial. JAMA Ophthalmol. 2014;132(7):866–73. https://doi.org/10.1001/jamaophthalmol.2014.1634. PMID: 24805262; PMCID: PMC4795002.
109. Park UC, Park JH, Ma DJ, Cho IH, Oh BL, Yu HG. A randomized paired-eye trial of intravitreal dexamethasone implant for cystoid macular edma in retinitis pigmentosa. Retina. 2020;40(7):1359–66. https://doi.org/10.1097/IAE.0000000000002589. PMID: 31166248.
110. Kumar A, Midha N, Gogia V, Gupta S, Sehra S, Chohan A. Efficacy of oral valproic acid in patients with retinitis pigmentosa. J Ocul Pharmacol Ther. 2014;30(7):580–6. https://doi.org/10.1089/jop.2013.0166. Epub 2014 Jun 23. PMID: 24955739.
111. Schatz A, Pach J, Gosheva M, Naycheva L, Willmann G, Wilhelm B, Peters T, Bartz-Schmidt KU, Zrenner E, Messias A, Gekeler F. Transcorneal electrical stimulation for patients with retinitis pigmentosa: a prospective, randomized, sham-controlled follow-up study over 1 year. Invest Ophthalmol Vis Sci. 2017;58(1):257–69. https://doi.org/10.1167/iovs.16-19906. PMID: 28114587.

Index

J. N. Weiss, *Clinical Trials in Retinitis Pigmentosa Treatment*,
https://doi.org/10.1007/978-3-031-58799-3

GPSR Compliance

The European Union's (EU) General Product Safety Regulation (GPSR) is a set of rules that requires consumer products to be safe and our obligations to ensure this.

If you have any concerns about our products, you can contact us on ProductSafety@springernature.com

In case Publisher is established outside the EU, the EU authorized representative is:

Springer Nature Customer Service Center GmbH
Europaplatz 3
69115 Heidelberg, Germany

Batch number: 10726135

Printed by Printforce, the Netherlands